T0013122

THE FIRST-TIME MOM'S PREGNANCY COOKBOOK

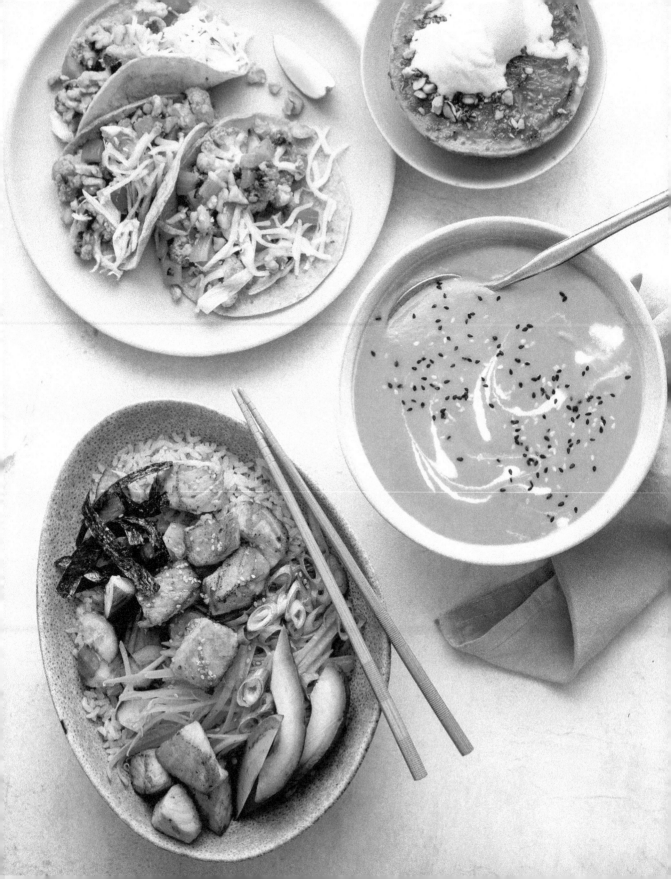

The First-Time Mom's Pregnancy Cookbook

A Nutrition Guide, Recipes, and
Meal Plans for a Healthy Pregnancy

Lauren Manaker, MS, RDN, LDN, CLEC, CPT
with additional recipes from Madeline Given

Photography by Annie Martin

ROCKRIDGE
PRESS

Interior and Cover Designer: Michael Cook
Art Producer: Hannah Dickerson
Editor: Claire Yee
Production Editor: Nora Milman
Production Manager: Michael Kay

Photography © 2021 Annie Martin, food styling by Nadine Page, cover and back cover (second from top, third from top) and pp. II, VI-VII, X, 24, 56, 96, 131, 157, 167; © Marija Vidal, back cover (top, bottom) and pp. 35, 39, 83, 89, 91, 119, 129, 138; iStock.com, p. 18. Decorative pattern used under license from Shutterstock.com. Author photo courtesy of Lydia Hunter. Recipe developer photo courtesy of Annemarie Bollman.

Cover: Kitchen Sink Kale Salad, page 75

ISBN: Print 978-1-64876-709-8 | eBook 978-1-64876-710-4
R0

This book is dedicated to all the expecting families who are embarking on the most rewarding and selfless journey of pregnancy and parenthood. I wish you joy and love during this magical time.

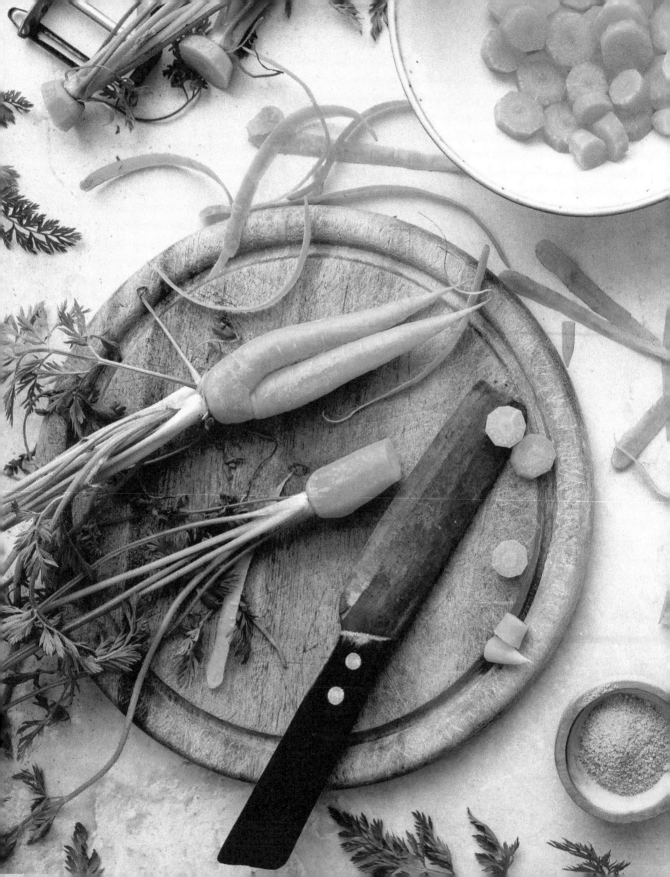

CONTENTS

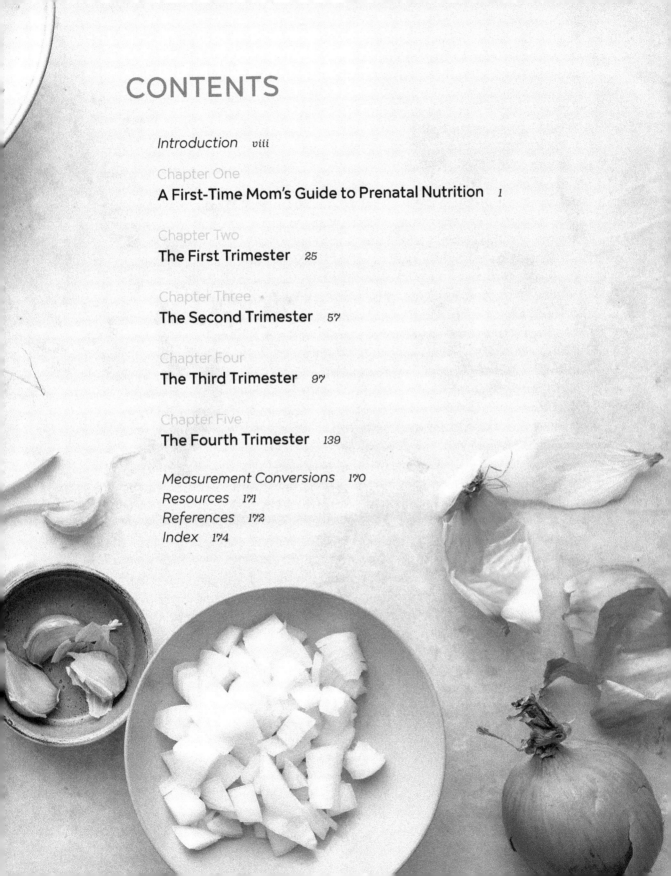

INTRODUCTION

Learning that you are expecting for the first time can come with a slew of emotions. During pregnancy, it is not unheard of to feel excitement one minute and complete and utter panic the next. Pregnancy is a special time in a person's life, but unfortunately it is also a time when unsolicited advice can come at you in full force, especially when it comes to nutrition. Between social media, Dr. Google, and your well-meaning and ever-knowing aunt, prenatal information overload can be very real and very overwhelming. With so much nutrition advice floating around, how do you know which advice to follow and which to pass by?

As a registered dietitian and a mother, I have seen firsthand how much conflicting nutrition information is offered. Trying to find the right nutrition guidance when you are eating for two can be dizzying, and there is a need for a guide that cuts through the fluff and highlights only evidence-based suggestions. I have made it my mission to dig into the available nutrition research to provide accurate information that expecting mothers need to have. Therefore, the information found in this book is based on data, not based off theory or a hunch. Nutrition plays a critical role in fetal development, and the guidance you will receive as a result from the most up-to-date research will help fuel your first pregnancy in a nourishing way that will benefit both you and your baby. No gimmicks, just science.

Nutrition is the cornerstone to health. Rest assured that reading this book will help ease any concerns you may have about food choices during pregnancy. You can clear out all the conflicting and overwhelming advice you have heard in the past and follow the simple steps that are provided in this book.

I wrote this book from the perspective of an award-winning nutrition expert with almost 20 years of experience who has experienced pregnancy firsthand. This book will demystify prenatal nutrition and provide some tips that are easy and realistic to implement. As a bonus, you will have access to some pregnancy-fueling recipes and sample meal plans that will help nourish your little one for the next nine months. Having this book in your back pocket will equip you to navigate your meals and snack choices confidently. I would like to personally welcome you on your pregnancy nutrition journey and am thrilled to be partnering with you.

HOW TO USE THIS BOOK

When you are pregnant, having a guide that acts as both a resource chock-full of nutrition information and a recipe book can be extremely useful, and that is exactly how this book is structured. You can read this book from cover to cover in one sitting or flip ahead to your particular pregnancy month.

The overall structure of this book is created to coincide with your journey and is broken down accordingly:

Chapter 1 offers general pregnancy nutrition information that mothers-to-be should have access to, but unfortunately don't always receive. It also includes important nutrient and food lists as well as practical advice for eating well and safely while pregnant.

Chapters 2 to 5 include targeted nutritional information to address different stages of pregnancy as well as the postpartum stage. These chapters are divided into trimesters, with a fourth trimester covering postpartum nutrition.

Included in these trimester chapters is not only important information, but also sample weekly meal plans for each month and delicious recipes for breakfast, lunch, dinner, and snack time that are rich in healthy nutrients for baby and mom. Each recipe is marked with its corresponding labels: Dairy-Free, Gluten-Free, Nut-Free, Vegetarian, and Freezer-Friendly. Additionally, you will find recipe tips to customize dishes for common pregnancy discomforts (we're looking at you, constipation) and personal preferences.

This book is an informational resource, recipe book, and meal planning guide all in one. It will surely be a great source of guidance for you to lean on during these special and important months.

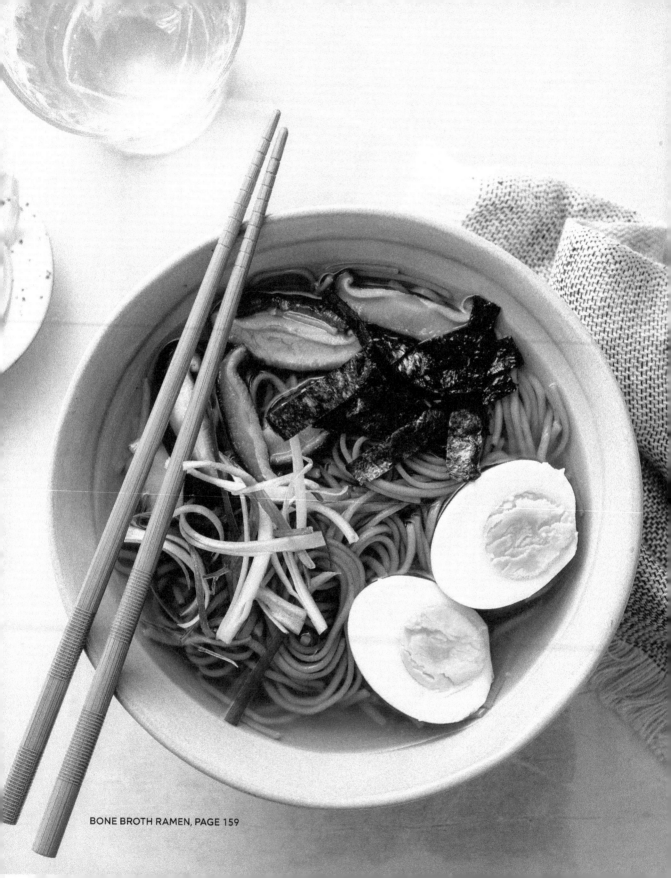

BONE BROTH RAMEN, PAGE 159

A First-Time Mom's Guide to Prenatal Nutrition

A pregnant mother's diet can play a role in her future baby's health for the rest of their lifetime. Eating to support a healthy pregnancy is not hard with the right know-how. The foods you choose should not potentially harm your baby, should ideally contain nutrients that offer some benefit to yourself or your baby, and most importantly, should taste good. Eating for two may look a little different than how you have been eating, but I promise it's simple—everything you need to know about nutrition as a first-time mom is right here in these pages.

Eating Well for Two

As a prenatal dietitian, the first questions I get asked by pregnant people are most often surrounding what they *can't* eat. It is unfortunate that many people are told all about the laundry list of foods they should avoid while they are pregnant, but they aren't informed on which foods they *should* be eating. Yes, there are some foods that should be avoided (if you're a ceviche or rare hamburger lover, you'll need to hold off on these foods while pregnant). But the focus should be more on which nutrients to eat during pregnancy to ensure that mama and baby are being fueled in the most optimal way.

Eating during pregnancy does not need to be complicated and filled with trendy foods like goji berries or maca. The focus should be on a balanced approach that's rich in nutrient-dense foods. These should pack a punch when it comes to certain pregnancy-fueling nutrients like protein, healthy fats, iron, folate, and choline. Contrary to what some people will tell you, there is no one pregnancy "superfood" that you must eat every day. Instead, eating a variety of foods from different food groups is key—that includes sweets! Believe it or not, even an occasional donut or "unhealthy" craving is perfectly fine to enjoy while you are expecting and won't harm your baby. The next few pages will dive into what the nutritional building blocks are for your first-time pregnancy.

Nutritional Building Blocks of a Healthy, Happy Pregnancy

Before we dive into what particular foods to eat and enjoy during your pregnancy, let's take a look at the nutritional foundation you'll create over these nine months.

Calories

Calorie needs increase during pregnancy. It takes a lot of energy to grow a human, and extra calories support this feat. Carrying multiples will require even more calories. Caloric intake should increase by about 300 calories per day during pregnancy and include nutrient-dense foods (not a daily dose of chocolate chip cookies). However, energy requirements are generally the same as those for non-pregnant people in the first trimester and then increase in the second and

WHAT TO KNOW ABOUT
PRENATAL VITAMINS AND SUPPLEMENTS

While eating a balanced diet can supply your body with important and pregnancy-fueling nutrients, you may require additional supplementation to meet the recommended nutrition needs required to support a healthy pregnancy. Prenatal vitamins can ensure that your body is supplied with key nutrients that you may not get in adequate amounts every single day via food. It is suggested to start taking a prenatal vitamin at least three months before conception, but if that isn't the case for you, it's never too late to start!

Prenatal vitamin needs vary based on your diet, lifestyle, and health status. For example, a person who follows a vegan lifestyle is likely going to require supplementation of different nutrients than a person who includes animal products in their meals. While it is always best to receive personalized supplementation advice, there are some general guidelines for supplement selection. The following are considerations that should minimally be taken in when selecting prenatal vitamins:

- At least 600mcg folic acid (methylated folate can be chosen as an alternative)
- At least 150mcg iodine in the form of potassium iodide
- At least 200mg DHA omega-3 fatty acids
- Supplemental choline depending on the person's dietary intake
- Vitamin D if not exposed to adequate natural sunlight
- Vitamin B_{12} and zinc, especially if a person follows a vegetarian or vegan lifestyle
- Calcium, especially if avoiding dairy and/or other calcium-rich foods

Supplemental iron may be required, especially during the second and third trimesters. It is important to note that many gummy prenatal vitamins do not contain iron. Vitamin C supplements (in doses around 200mg) can assist with iron absorption, while milk and tea can inhibit iron supplementation.

Some pregnant people may also benefit from:

- A probiotic supplement to help maintain healthy bowel movements or possibly reduce the risk of the baby having eczema
- Vitamin B_6 to help alleviate nausea
- Choline if the 450mg daily intake requirement is not met
- Additional iron if iron-deficient
- Carnitine to possibly reduce the risk of developing gestational diabetes
- Magnesium to possibly help relieve leg cramps

Consult with your health care provider for guidance.

third trimesters, estimated at 340 calories and 452 calories per day, respectively. Calorie needs can vary depending on a pregnant person's age, pre-pregnancy weight, activity level, health status, and other factors.

Macronutrients

Calories come in the form of macronutrients: carbohydrates, protein, and fat. All three of these macronutrients serve important roles in a pregnant person's body. So, unless your doctor explicitly tells you otherwise, you should make a point to eat a diet that is composed of all three of these nutrients. We will dig into specifics surrounding each macronutrient later in this chapter.

Micronutrients

Micronutrients include vitamins and minerals, and some play an extremely pivotal role in prenatal health. Some key nutrients for a healthy pregnancy include:

Calcium. This nutrient is found in foods with dairy such as cheese, milk, and yogurt. It helps strengthen baby's developing bones. Not enough calcium intake during pregnancy, especially during the third trimester, can lead to osteoporosis and brittle bones.

Choline. This nutrient is found in egg yolks, peanuts, and cauliflower. It plays an important role in baby's brain development and may be protective against certain birth defects. It is estimated that 90 percent of Americans are not meeting the estimated needs of choline, and most prenatal vitamins do not contain any of this brain-boosting nutrient.

DHA. This omega-3 fatty acid is found in many seafood choices like salmon and shrimp. It is also found in algae. Adequate maternal DHA intake is linked to positive outcomes for baby's brain and eye development, among other benefits. Some moms with high DHA levels during pregnancy may experience longer pregnancies and fewer preterm births.

Folate. This B vitamin is found in avocado, green leafy vegetables, and beets. Folate has been shown to reduce the risk of babies developing certain birth defects like spina bifida, which affects the baby's spinal cord. Folic acid is the synthetic form of the vitamin and needs to be converted to folate to be utilized. If you have a suspected or known challenge making this conversion, then supplements made with folate, methylated folate, or MTHF folate should be chosen.

Iodine. Found in foods like cod, nori seaweed, and iodized salt, this nutrient is important for baby's brain development and needs to be increased during pregnancy. Too much iodine can pose risks during pregnancy, so this is one nutrient to not oversupplement.

Iron. This nutrient is found in foods like red meats, crab, and green leafy vegetables. A pregnant person's blood volume doubles during pregnancy, especially as their belly size increases. Iron helps build new red blood cells that carry oxygen throughout their body and to their baby. Not getting enough iron can result in fatigue as well as more severe outcomes like preterm birth.

Vitamin A. While there is data that suggests consuming excessive amounts of preformed vitamin A during pregnancy can cause potential harm to the fetus, adequate amounts of this nutrient are important for proper development of baby's organs and skeleton, among other benefits. Foods that are naturally orange in color like pumpkin and carrots are rich in beta-carotene, which the body converts to vitamin A. Milk is a source of preformed vitamin A.

Vitamin D. This fat-soluble vitamin plays an important role in pregnancy, and deficiency may be linked to baby's risk of developing type 1 diabetes, among other outcomes. Foods that contain vitamin D include salmon, dairy milk, fortified nondairy alternatives, and egg yolks. It is advised to get your vitamin D levels checked to ensure you don't have any deficiency during pregnancy and to supplement accordingly.

Ensuring your diet contains a variety of macronutrients and micronutrients is key to having a healthy pregnancy. Your baby depends on your intake to get what it needs to grow and develop, so touching on all the important nutrients is essential. For a more detailed look at the daily requirements of micronutrients during pregnancy, see the Key Micronutrients chart (page 10).

Foods to Enjoy

So now we know that a balanced diet rich in variety is key when pregnant. But, specifically, which foods are great choices for a pregnancy, which should be limited, and which are a no-go? Let's break down some foods by category to help you navigate your plate.

Whole Grains

Carbohydrate intake is one topic that you don't want to lean on social media for advice. Some self-proclaimed nutrition experts will lead you to believe that carbohydrates of any kind should be eliminated, no matter what.

Carbohydrates fuel your body with important energy, can be a source of fiber, and can be a great source of important vitamins, minerals, and antioxidants. Cutting them out of your diet may pose a risk. However, not all carbohydrates are created equal.

One group of carbohydrates that you want to include in your pregnancy diet is whole grains. Some people opt to follow a grain-free diet or a gluten-free diet for personal health reasons. Keep in mind that some whole grains like corn (including popcorn) and quinoa are gluten-free.

Whole grains include grains eaten in the *whole* form. Hence the name *whole* grains! Some examples of whole grains include:

Barley	Quinoa	Sorghum
Corn	Rice	Spelt
Oats	Rye	Wheat

Whole grains should replace refined grains like white rice, white bread, and white flour. Brown rice, whole grain bread, and 100 percent whole grain flour are great swaps. Whole grains provide the ever-important fiber into your diet, which will help keep bowel movements healthy and keep you feeling full for a longer period of time. Foods like white rice have the natural fiber removed, while brown rice retains this important nutrient.

Antioxidants are needed in higher amounts during pregnancy to combat the oxidative stress that naturally occurs. Whole grains are naturally rich in antioxidants, as well as other key pregnancy-fueling nutrients like certain B vitamins, magnesium, and iron. Additionally, the carbohydrates in whole grains digest more slowly when compared with more refined carbs, and therefore help the body avoid a blood sugar spike and potential crash later on. The nutrients found in whole grains benefit baby as well. Many whole grains are fortified with nutrients like folic acid, a key nutrient to support baby's development.

Whole grains are simple to sneak into your diet. Enjoy a sandwich on slices of 100 percent whole grain bread, snack on some homemade popcorn, or eat your stir-fry over a bed of quinoa instead of white rice.

Healthy Fats

Fats should not be avoided. Instead, they should be chosen wisely. When you choose to eat the right kind of fat, you are fueling your body to support your baby's brain development, of which 60 percent is made of fat. Many foods that are rich in healthy fats are also rich in important fat-soluble vitamins like vitamins A, D, E, and K—nutrients that support a healthy pregnancy and help maximize absorption of other vitamins. However, eating too much fat, no matter of which type, is linked to some undesired outcomes for your baby. So, eat your fat—just don't overdo it.

The fats that should be emphasized are the unsaturated varieties, and trans fats should be avoided. Foods like avocado, nuts, and plant-based oils like olive oil are excellent choices for a pregnancy-supporting diet. Foods like prepackaged pastries, many coffee creamers, and vegetable shortenings often contain trans fats and are not the best choice for this stage in life.

One key healthy fat to consume during pregnancy is a specific omega-3 fatty acid called docosahexaenoic acid, or DHA. This fatty acid is mostly found in marine animals like certain fish and shellfish. It is also found in some fortified foods, such as milk and orange juice. Additionally, certain eggs contain DHA if the chickens are fed food containing DHA. This fatty acid has been shown to support baby's brain and eye health and may even reduce the risk of mom developing postpartum depression.

Fruits and Vegetables

Eating a wide variety of fruits and vegetables is one of the best things you can do for yourself and your baby when you are pregnant. These foods offer a slew of benefits that can't be replicated by supplements.

Fiber is a pregnant person's best friend while experiencing the common side effect of constipation. As certain hormone levels rise in pregnancy, the intestinal muscles relax, and bowel movements don't happen as easily. Additionally, the pressure of the expanding uterus onto the intestines can contribute to a backed-up feeling. Many fruits and vegetables are naturally rich in fiber. Just make sure to keep the skin on choices like cucumber, apple, and sweet potato to get the most bang for your fiber buck.

Proteins

Protein needs increase during pregnancy and help support both baby's growth and development as well as mom's personal needs. Protein is found in foods like meats, eggs, nuts, tofu, and beans. Recommended protein intake during pregnancy is 60g/day, which represents an increase from 46g/day in non-pregnant states.

Most of the proteins that you choose should be lean sources—think fish, meats without visible fat, and eggs. Lean proteins are lower in saturated fats. They are also oftentimes lower in calories, but still fuel a pregnant body with protein along with important nutrients like vitamin B_{12}, iron, and zinc in certain cases. While more fatty cuts of meats should be limited, know that certain amino acids are needed in higher amounts during pregnancy and these are found in connective tissue and the skin of meat. Therefore, incorporating some chicken or fish with the skin on, meats on the bone, and even baked pork rinds can offer some benefit to a pregnant mother if consumed in moderation.

If you live a vegetarian or vegan lifestyle, it is important to include lean nonmeat proteins in your diet. Beans, peas, and lentils are all plant-based protein sources that are satisfying and nutritious. Note that these choices are low in a few essential amino acids. Eating a variety of other foods can help fill in gaps. Nuts are another plant-based protein source that is a good complement to beans, peas, and lentils. If you include dairy in your diet, a glass of milk can provide your body with important amino acids, too.

Dairy and Nondairy Sources of Calcium

Around 1,000mg of calcium a day is necessary to support mama and baby's bones, teeth, and other organs. Calcium also helps support heart health and is important for muscle function. Dairy foods like milk, yogurt, and cottage cheese are excellent sources of calcium and contain other nutrients like protein, vitamin D, and vitamin A. It is suggested to consume two to three servings of dairy daily while pregnant.

If you avoid dairy for whatever reason, calcium can easily be obtained by other food sources like tofu, green leafy vegetables, and almonds. Dairy alternatives like oat milk are often fortified with this important mineral. If you are avoiding dairy foods, it is important for the expecting mother to be conscious about calcium intake and supplement accordingly if their needs are not being met through diet.

Fish and Shellfish

Seafood is one of the best sources of unique fatty acids: DHA and EPA. These have been linked to supporting baby's brain and eye development, reduced risk of mom developing postpartum depression, and better attention spans in pre-school children.

Fish and shellfish should be a part of a pregnancy diet, with some caveats. Seafood can contain levels of toxic metals, specifically mercury. Pregnant mothers who take in too much mercury put their baby at risk for some negative outcomes. The key is to take in enough seafood to fuel mom with enough important DHA, EPA, and other nutrients like protein and selenium, while not taking in too much.

Certain seafood choices have been shown to contain less mercury when compared to others. In general, the larger fish that prey on smaller fish contain higher mercury levels—think shark, swordfish, and marlin. Seafood lower in the food chain, like shrimp, scallops, and tilapia, are better choices.

Typically, two (four-ounce) servings of low-mercury seafood is recommended. DHA supplements should be takin in conjunction with the twice-weekly seafood intake to ensure mom is taking in enough DHA.

KEY MICRONUTRIENTS

KEY NUTRIENT	DAILY REQUIREMENTS FOR PREGNANCY/ LACTATION	WHAT THIS NUTRIENT DOES	FOODS RICH IN THIS NUTRIENT
VITAMIN A	Pregnancy: 770mcg RAE (retinol activity equivalent) Extremely high doses of retinol supplements aren't recommended during this time. Lactation: 1,200mcg RAE for lactation	Supports baby's eye health and mom and baby's immune health	Retinol: Animal fats, liver, cod liver oil Beta-carotene: many naturally orange foods like carrots, sweet potatoes, apricot, cantaloupe, dark green leafy greens
VITAMIN B$_9$ (FOLATE)	Pregnancy: 600mcg DFE (dietary folate equivalent) Lactation: 500mcg DFE	Reduces baby's risk of developing certain birth defects, promotes DNA and cell production, and reduces risk of baby developing cleft palate.	Green leafy vegetables, beets, avocados, citrus, nuts, seeds, and strawberries
CHOLINE	Pregnancy: 450mg Lactation: 550mg	Recognized as a "brain-building" nutrient, may improve cognitive function in your baby into adulthood, and play a role in neural tube development.	Beef, egg yolks, chicken, fish, pork, nuts, peanuts, and cruciferous vegetables, such as broccoli and cauliflower
DHA	Pregnancy and lactation: 20+ mg	Helps with growth and development. Critical for fetal neurodevelopment and helps in developing the brain, eyes, liver, fat, and skeletal muscle.	Seafoods that are low in mercury, such as herring, scallops, salmon, anchovies, and halibut. Orange juice, milk, and eggs that have DHA added to them. If a person is avoiding seafood, they can opt for an algae-based DHA supplement.

KEY NUTRIENT	DAILY REQUIREMENTS FOR PREGNANCY/ LACTATION	WHAT THIS NUTRIENT DOES	FOODS RICH IN THIS NUTRIENT
IODINE	Pregnancy: 220mcg to 290mcg Lactation: 290mcg Supplements should contain at least 150mcg/ day of iodine. Potassium iodide is the preferred source of iodine for prenatal vitamins.	Essential for healthy brain development in the fetus and young child. Low iodide can lead to low thyroid levels, which can be associated with complications during pregnancy, like poor fetal growth, preterm birth, and miscarriage.	Use iodized salt when cooking. Roasted nori seaweed snacks, cod.
CALCIUM	Pregnancy and Lactation: 1,000mg If you are pregnant at 18 years old or younger, you need 1,300mg. Taking high amounts of calcium with iron is not advised, as both nutrients may compete for absorption in the body. If supplementing, do not take more than 500mg calcium at a time.	Helps strengthen baby's developing bones and boosts muscle, heart, and nerve development.	Foods with dairy, such as cheese, milk, and yogurt. Dark green leafy vegetables and legumes, like broccoli, Brussels sprouts, collards, kale, mustard greens, and tofu. Foods with calcium added to them, like orange juices and cereals.
IRON	Pregnancy: 27mg Needs often do not increase until second trimester. Lactation: 9mg However, if there was a lot of blood loss during labor, a person may need more iron. Once a mother starts menstruating, her needs will likely increase.	Supports your baby's developing blood supply with healthy red blood cells, prevents anemia in you and your baby, and helps deliver an appropriate amount of oxygen to your growing body as well as the baby. Encourages proper fetal brain development.	Heme iron (found in meat): beef, chicken, eggs, canned sardines. Non-heme iron (found in vegetables): white beans, lentils, spinach, cashews, and even dark chocolate!
VITAMIN D	Pregnancy and lactation: 600 IU minimum If supplementing, D_3 is the preferred form of this vitamin, as opposed to vitamin D_2.	Plays an important role in immune function and bone health, may prevent preterm birth, and reduces risk of baby developing cavities later in life.	Certain fish, milk, fortified milk alternatives, and egg yolk.

Foods to Watch Out For

Eating a wide variety of nutrient-dense foods is recommended during pregnancy. But there are some foods that should be eaten with caution or avoided altogether to help keep you and your baby safe.

Caffeine

Caffeine is found in drinks like coffee, certain teas, chocolate, matcha, kombucha, and energy drinks. It has been shown to cross the placenta and excessive amounts have been linked to miscarriage risk in some studies (not all). Experts recommend keeping caffeine intake below 200 to 300mg per day. Some people will opt for decaffeinated coffee as a caffeine-free swap from coffee. Decaffeinated coffee is not caffeine-free. If you plan to drink decaf, do some research on the brand you choose to know how much caffeine you are actually taking in.

CBD

Many people swear by cannabidiol, often referred to as CBD, and are in the habit of ingesting it regularly. Unfortunately, there is not enough data to know whether CBD is safe to ingest during pregnancy. For this reason, it is suggested that pregnant people err on the side of caution and avoid CBD-containing foods and drinks.

Alcohol

No amount of alcohol has been established to offer any benefit to your baby during pregnancy. While some may argue that small amounts of alcohol exposure cause no harm to the baby, data suggests that even a small amount of alcohol exposure can pose harm. Mocktails can be your go-to drink for the next few months. If you opt for a booze-free beer, know that some brands contain a small amount of alcohol, so do your homework on brands. If you regularly add a splash of red wine to your pasta sauce or bake with real brandy, know that heat from cooking "cooks off" the alcohol. Foods like rum raisin ice cream are often perfectly safe as well.

Other Beverages

Smoothies can be a lifesaver if you're experiencing nausea and can't stomach vegetables any other way. Just be mindful of any added juices, because unpasteurized options can pose a health risk. Protein powders are a common addition to some recipes, and in some cases are a great and safe choice. However, some protein powder options are not the best for pregnancy, because they contain additional ingredients that have the potential to cause harm. When choosing protein powder, make sure it does not contain components like a laundry list of ingredients, including some fillers. Avoid any herbs, artificial ingredients, or high amounts of added vitamins. Single-ingredient protein powders are often your best bet.

Some teas should be limited or avoided during pregnancy. Black, oolong, and matcha naturally contain caffeine. If you are limiting your caffeine intake, these teas should count toward your quota for the day. Some herbal teas, such as motherwort, fenugreek, and fennel, should be avoided during pregnancy, because they may increase risk of miscarriage or birth defects. On the other hand, teas made from real fruits or ginger tea are great choices while expecting.

There are some concerns surrounding kombucha and pregnancy. Kombucha contains a small amount of alcohol as an effect of the fermentation, is often not pasteurized, and is often made with caffeinated tea. Experts appear to be on the fence when it comes to this beverage during pregnancy. To err on the safe side, skip it until your baby is here. If you must have kombucha, opt for a caffeine-free or pasteurized option. Just know that if it is pasteurized, the live and beneficial bacteria is often killed off in the process and is therefore ineffective.

Raw or Undercooked Seafood and Meat

Eating low-mercury fish and seafood is an important part of a pregnancy diet. However, raw or undercooked seafood should be avoided when you are pregnant. The illnesses of greatest concern from eating raw or undercooked clams or oysters are vibrio, norovirus, and hepatitis A—all conditions that you definitely do not want to experience when you are expecting.

Likewise, raw or undercooked meat should be avoided during pregnancy. Eating it increases the risk of being exposed to salmonella and E. coli bacteria, as well as other exposures that can cause foodborne illness. Stick with well-cooked meat to play it safe. The inside of your chicken and beef should not be pink.

Seafood with Higher Mercury

Seafood that is higher on the food chain should be avoided due to concerns of mercury ingestion. Some fish that should be avoided during pregnancy include swordfish, shark, king mackerel, and bluefish tuna. Stick to the low-mercury options and aim for two servings per week.

Canned skipjack is considered to be a "low-mercury" choice and can be enjoyed during pregnancy. Albacore tuna should be limited to 6 ounces per week. Tuna is an excellent source of DHA omega-3 fatty acids, is a high-quality protein, and contains pregnancy-fueling nutrients such as iodine, selenium, and vitamin B_{12}. When choosing canned tuna, try to pick varieties that guarantee no BPA in the lining of the can—or better yet, choose a shelf-stable tuna pouch option to avoid BPA exposure risk altogether.

Deli Meat

You don't have to give up deli meats completely when you are pregnant, as long as you take some precautionary steps. While the risk is low, consuming deli meats may put a pregnant mom at risk for a foodborne illness called listeria, which could be quite dangerous during pregnancy. But if you can't do without them, keep these tips in mind:

Heat your deli meat in the microwave before you eat it or make a toasted or pressed sandwich with the meat thoroughly heated.

Don't consume any deli meat that looks or tastes questionable.

Be mindful of expiration dates and ensure that your deli meat is stored at safe temperatures.

When possible, choose fresher meats like turkey off the bone.

Choose lower-sodium options of deli meats and opt for those that are not loaded with fillers or additives.

Undercooked Eggs

Eating undercooked eggs puts you at risk for salmonella poisoning, which could be extremely dangerous when pregnant. Choose fully cooked eggs—think scrambled or hard-boiled—or purchase pasteurized eggs to ensure your safety. Be wary of foods like hollandaise sauce, Caesar dressing, and homemade ice cream, all of which can be made with raw/unpasteurized egg.

Unpasteurized Dairy, Juices, and Honey

Pasteurization kills potentially harmful bacteria. Unfortunately, it's not a step that is always taken in juice bars. Read your labels, ask questions, or better yet, stick with a piece of whole fruit instead of the juiced version. The same rule applies to unpasteurized cheese.

Honey in moderation can be a part of a healthy pregnancy diet as long as it is pasteurized honey. If you are buying your honey from a roadside stand, chances are it is not pasteurized. You will see an indication on the label.

Unwashed Produce

Wash your produce well before enjoying. Many fruits and vegetables go through many channels before they reach your kitchen and that means many opportunities for contamination. Yes, that includes washing the rinds of melons before cutting into them—even though you don't eat it, bacteria can reach the "meat" of the melon when you are cutting through the rind.

Raw Sprouts and Mushrooms

Alfalfa, radish, clover, and mung bean sprouts are some examples of sprout varieties that should be avoided during pregnancy. Although they offer a refreshing crunch when added to salads and sandwiches, they are a high-risk food for containing bacteria that could make you very sick.

Any type of "magic mushrooms" should be off-limits for the next nine months (and probably for a while after baby arrives as well). Mushrooms purchased at the grocery store are fine to eat, but make sure that you only eat cooked mushrooms while you are eating for two to reduce the risk of health issues.

Raw Cookie Dough

Whether or not raw cookie dough is egg-free or made with raw eggs, it can still be dangerous to eat for pregnant people. The concern with raw cookie dough isn't always the eggs, but rather the flour. Raw flour can contain bacteria that can make you sick. For the next nine months, your best bet is to stick with good old-fashioned chocolate chip cookies (with milk!).

Real Black Licorice

Data suggests that consuming black licorice is linked to some negative outcomes, like high blood pressure for mom, a shorter pregnancy, and cognitive concerns for baby later on in life. If you are a red licorice fan, keep on giving into your sugar fix (in moderation). Just skip the black licorice for now. That goes for licorice tea, too!

Stay Hydrated!

Dehydration during pregnancy can potentially put your baby at risk. Because your body is gradually growing (hello, baby bump!), your body needs to take in more fluid to support the extra volume. Specifically, a lack of fluids during pregnancy increases risk for conditions like premature labor and low amniotic fluid. Even if you are not moving around much or sweating, you still need to maintain your hydration.

The Institute of Medicine recommends about 10 cups of fluids a day during pregnancy. A great rule of thumb is to drink before thirst is felt. A great indicator of hydration is checking your urine color—if it is deep yellow and concentrated, you likely need to drink more. Just note that some supplements may turn urine very yellow regardless of hydration status. You may also feel fatigue, have headaches, or feel dizzy if you are not adequately hydrated. Dehydration may also trigger Braxton-Hicks contractions, or uncomfortable false-labor pain.

To stay hydrated, carry a water bottle at all times, and drink often. While water is an excellent choice, explore other options like infused waters and seltzer for a little variety. Coconut water and maple water on occasion can be a welcome alternative that provides a little sweetness along with natural electrolytes. Also, don't forget that foods like watermelon are over 90 percent water, so you can always eat your fluids, too!

You can't judge a food by its box, but you **can** judge a food by its nutrition label. Nutrition labels provide insight into which nutrients the item contains. Using food labels can help you decide whether a food item is actually doing something good for your body.

One key aspect of a food label is the ingredient list. It's important to keep in mind that the ingredients are listed in order of which item is used most to which is used the least. Let's say you are comparing two jarred pasta sauces: One has sugar listed as the first ingredient and tomatoes as the sixth, while the second has tomatoes listed as a first ingredient and only has three ingredients listed. The second jar will likely be made with more nutrient-rich tomatoes and therefore would be a better choice.

Although there are many micronutrients that are important for pregnancy support, the FDA mandates that each food label lists the amount and percentage of daily recommended amounts of only four micronutrients: vitamin D, calcium, iron, and potassium. All four of these nutrients help support a healthy pregnancy. The absence of other vitamins and minerals listed on the food label does not mean that the food does not contain any of the nutrients. It is simply not required to be listed.

Eating Healthy Portions and a Balanced Plate

A healthy portion size for one person may not be the best amount of food for another. For example, a very active person who is pregnant with twins will likely require more calories, and therefore larger portion sizes, when compared with a person who is pregnant with only one baby and lives a more sedentary lifestyle. Keep in mind that a portion size is different from a serving size, which is a quantity that is indicated on the nutrition label and is a standard amount of food, like a cup or an ounce. Serving sizes are not recommendations for how much a person should eat.

In my practice, I like to recommend that portion sizes be kept on the smaller side to allow for a wide variety of food from different food groups. Here are suggested portion sizes of some popular foods:

3 ounces of poultry or meat—a deck of cards or the palm of a hand

3 ounces of fish—a checkbook

1 ounce of cheese—four dice

1 medium potato—a computer mouse

2 tablespoons of nut butter—a ping-pong ball

1 cup of pasta—a tennis ball

An ideal meal plate is composed of more than one food group in appropriate portion sizes. For example, instead of eating a large bowl of 2 to 3 cups of spaghetti with sauce for dinner, I would rather see a 1-cup serving of whole grain pasta topped with sauce and 3 ounces of grilled chicken with 1 cup of cooked broccoli tossed with 1 tablespoon of olive oil. A glass of milk as a beverage would round out this meal and provide a serving of food from various important food groups.

A healthy and balanced plate should ideally look like this:

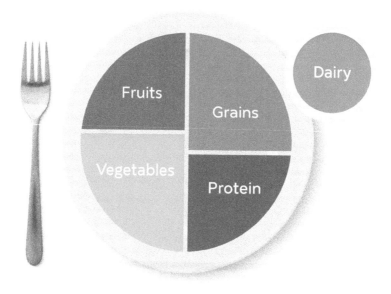

- One nonstarchy vegetable and one fruit serving, or two nonstarchy vegetable servings
- Whole grain starch or starchy vegetable like a sweet potato
- Protein source like meat, fish, or nuts
- Healthy plant oils like olive oils
- Beverages should consist mostly of water

In addition to the ideal plate, two to three servings of dairy foods should be enjoyed if the overall diet is low in calcium, and sweets can be enjoyed in a limited capacity. All these recommendations may vary based on your own individual needs and whether you are managing any conditions like gestational diabetes.

TRY NOT TO STRESS ABOUT WEIGHT GAIN

When growing another human being inside your body, it is healthy and necessary to gain weight. The additional weight will make up your baby's body mass, your placenta, additional fluid, and other factors. The Institute of Medicine provides recommendations for weight gain during pregnancy based on a person's pre-pregnancy body mass index, or BMI. To calculate your BMI, simply calculate your weight (in kilograms) divided by the square of your height (in meters). BMI = kg/m2.

The guidelines set forth by this institute in 2009 are as follows in the table below::

BODY MASS INDEX	RECOMMENDED RANGE OF TOTAL WEIGHT GAINED
Less than 18.5	28 to 40 pounds
18.5–24.9	25 to 35 pounds
25–29.9	15 to 25 pounds

Although BMI is used quite often in the medical world to assess how "healthy" a person's weight is, it's not a perfect tool and does not take into account factors like lean body mass (muscle mass), ethnicity, or overall health. This weight gain guide should be used in conjunction with looking at the big picture to determine how much weight you should gain during pregnancy. Gradual weight gain is advised, with the most weight gained during the second and third trimesters.

Your doctor will likely weigh you during every prenatal visit, and it is important to follow any guidance they may provide if you are gaining too little or too much weight. As long as you follow your doctor's advice, eat a generally healthy diet, and exercise, weight gain should not be a huge stress factor for you!

Eating to Alleviate Pesky Pregnancy Symptoms

There are some magical parts of pregnancy, and there are some not-so-great aspects. Some people experience zero negative pregnancy symptoms, and others get the "pleasure" of experiencing them all. If you don't feel any symptoms, that is not a sign that something is wrong. Just consider yourself lucky! There are some common side effects that can possibly be managed via diet, including nausea and food aversions, heartburn, constipation, and fatigue.

Nausea and Food Aversions

Nausea is very common, especially during the first trimester, although it sometimes carries over to the second trimester. Food aversions are more common in the second trimester. If you are too queasy to eat normally, know that your body has an amazing way of getting what it needs and relies on nutrient stores. Only in severe cases does taking in inadequate food affect the baby—if you fall into this category, you should lean on your doctor's advice. Some simple tips for managing pregnancy-induced nausea and food aversions include:

- Avoid strong smells and spices (like garlic).

- Keep fresh-cut slices of lemon in your bag and smell them if you catch a whiff of strong perfume that is going to put you over the top.

- Cook with fresh ginger, eat ginger candies, or sip on ginger ale made with real ginger (make sure to keep the daily intake below 1,000mg to keep baby safe and check food labels—many brands are made with ginger flavoring and in reality, contain zero ginger).

- Stick with bland foods like a baked potato, toast, and crackers.

- If your prenatal vitamin is not agreeing with you, consider temporarily taking a gummy version until you feel better.

- Discuss taking additional B_6 supplementation with your doctor.

- Sneak vegetables in via a smoothie or enjoy plain-cooked "easy" veggies like carrots.

Nausea and morning sickness can cause some stress to an expecting mother but be reassured that the temporary discomfort rarely results in any issues in baby's development. However, dehydration can be a cause of concern if adequate liquid is not being consumed. Make a point to stay hydrated by sipping on fluids like water, broth, coconut water, or even ginger ale made with real ginger. You should also continue to take a prenatal vitamin if you can tolerate it. If taking the supplement is a challenge, share this issue with your doctor to find a solution.

For a nausea-friendly recipe, try Grandma's Homemade Chicken Noodle Soup (page 51), Hydrating Watermelon Fruit Pops (page 55), Banana-Chia Pudding (page 40), Power-Packed Oats (page 38), and Nix the Nausea Smoothie (page 37).

Heartburn

Hormonal changes and baby pushing into digestive organs can cause heartburn, especially later in pregnancy. Although it is an annoying side effect, it is very common. Some tips for managing heartburn include:

- Sitting upright after meals

- Avoiding spicy food

- Avoiding spearmint, chocolate, citrus, and caffeine

- Drinking dairy milk

For some helpful recipes in avoiding heartburn, try Blueberry Baked Oatmeal (page 109), Ginger-Cauliflower Smoothie (page 36), Avocado and Sweet Potato Toast (page 72), Whipped Cottage Cheese Berry Bowl (page 68), or Banana Custard with Chia (page 111).

Constipation

Feeling backed up? Welcome to the club. Many pregnant people experience constipation—a result of hormones taking a toll on your digestive system and your baby pushing in places that slows down bowel movements. These hormones are responsible for many positive aspects of a healthy pregnancy, but having high levels circulate in the body may result in a relaxation of the muscles in your digestive system. Thankfully, you may find relief by trying the following remedies:

Eat fiber-rich foods. Aiming for a fiber intake of 25 to 35 grams per day is recommended during pregnancy and can easily be achieved by eating whole grains, fruits, vegetables, nuts, and seeds. If you are increasing your fiber, you also need to increase your fluid intake. If you don't keep your fill of fluids, your bowels can become backed up and you can have a difficult time trying to find constipation relief. Drinking fluids that are room temperature instead of ice cold has been shown to be more beneficial in some cases.

Get moving. Physical activity has been shown to help keep the bowels healthy and is a great addition to any prenatal regimen. An exercise plan does not need to be anything elaborate—simply walking 20 minutes per day three times a week can sometimes do the trick.

Try probiotics. These are live beneficial bacteria found in fermented foods like yogurt and kimchi that can help support a healthy gut, and in turn, support healthy bowel movements. Probiotic supplementation can be discussed with your doctor as an alternative.

As a last resort, consult with your doctor about suppositories. This option should be discussed with your doctor and should not be abused.

For some helpful recipes in battling constipation heartburn, try Date with a Smoothie (page 112), Chicken with Dates (page 122), Walnut Tacos (page 121), Roasted Cauliflower Salad (page 117), or Crispy Chili Chickpeas (page 135).

Fatigue

Growing a human plus limited caffeine equals a recipe for exhaustion. Energy drinks or getting a quick caffeine jolt aren't the best options right now, but there are some ways to help combat pregnancy-induced fatigue, including:

Take a nap when timing allows, and don't feel guilty about it!

Eat complex carbohydrates and avoid very sugary foods like candies.

Eat breakfast regularly.

Exercise, even if it is a short stroll.

For some helpful recipes in fighting fatigue, try Maple-Quinoa Bark (page 94), Peanut Butter Fruit Dip with Sliced Apples (page 92), Mediterranean-Inspired Stuffed Sweet Potatoes (page 78), Super Spiced Choco-Latte (page 67), or Sweet Potato Pancakes (page 69).

Celebrate Progress, Not Perfection

Pregnancy and parenting can be emotionally exhausting. Now's a great time to strengthen a healthy and self-compassionate perspective on life. Not every day will be made of healthy greens and an invigorating yoga session. Some days may instead call for a lazy day on the couch along with a delivery from your local pizzeria. Don't forget to ask for support from others—this is a big task! Make sure to practice self-compassion and follow your body's cues, and as long as you are focusing on the big picture, you will be doing just fine, mama. If you ever find yourself backtracking and eating less than healthily a few days in a row, come back to these meal plans and recipes in the next chapters. You've got this, and this book is here to help!!

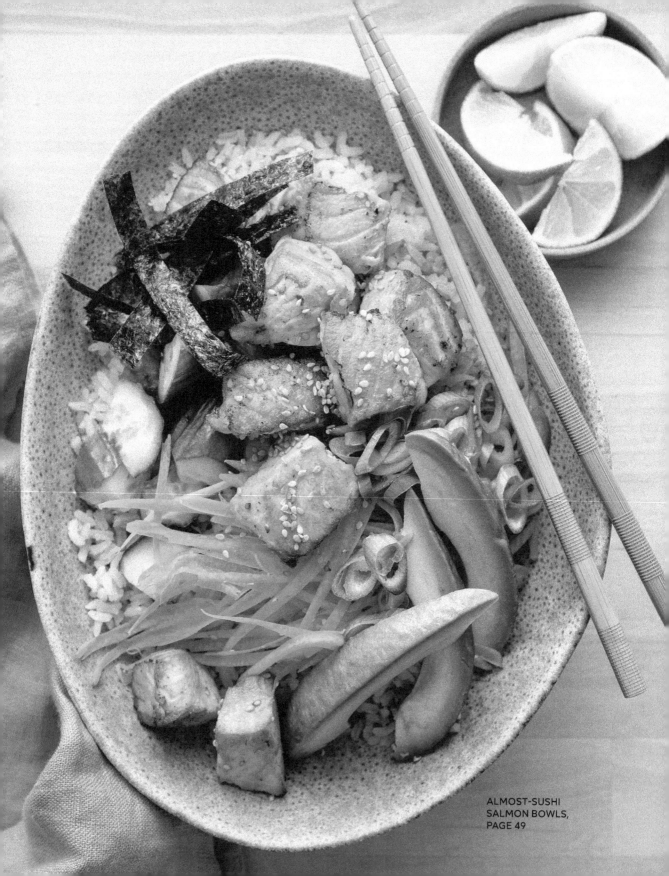

ALMOST-SUSHI
SALMON BOWLS,
PAGE 49

CHAPTER TWO
The First Trimester

Welcome to your first trimester and the beginning of the pregnancy journey. Although the first three months of pregnancy can come with some excitement and that radiant pregnancy glow, it can also come with some unwelcomed side effects (I'm looking at you, morning sickness). Just know that many symptoms are temporary and only mean that your body is responding to the natural hormonal changes that come with pregnancy.

Month 1: From Period to Pregnant

During the first month of pregnancy, your body will release certain hormones that will help support your pregnancy. Unfortunately, these hormones may also cause some PMS-like symptoms such as mood swings and exhaustion. Unless you are underweight, you will likely not need to increase your caloric intake at this early stage of pregnancy. Your focus should be on the baby's need for certain nutrients to support its neural tube development this month: folic acid or folate, choline, and vitamin B_{12}.

Fortified foods like cereals and certain breads contain folic acid. Folate is found naturally in foods like green leafy vegetables, beets, and avocados. The body converts folic acid into folate, the form of this nutrient that the body uses to perform its various roles. Data suggests that adequate folic acid intake helps reduce the risk of neural tube defects and cleft palate.

Choline is a nutrient that has been shown to support the healthy development of baby's neural tube, and therefore helps reduce the risk of baby developing certain birth defects. As discussed earlier, choline is not found in most prenatal vitamins. Egg yolks are one of the best sources of choline. Foods like peanuts, chicken, salmon, and cauliflower contain choline as well.

Vitamin B_{12} is the third nutrient that should be focused on during the first month of pregnancy. In conjunction with folic acid and choline, this B vitamin helps support baby's neural tube development as well. Foods that contain vitamin B_{12} include meats, nutritional yeast, salmon, and milk.

Now is a good time to stop drinking alcohol, smoking cigarettes, or taking any recreational drugs. You should also try to keep your caffeine intake below 200mg per day. Typically, one cup of coffee per day is under this amount. To stay on the safe side, avoiding caffeine altogether eliminates any caffeine-related complications during pregnancy, including the risk of miscarriage.

WHAT TO EXPECT THIS MONTH

How Baby Is Developing: The sperm and the egg meet, and your pregnancy journey begins. The embryo implants into the uterus and is in the beginning stages of becoming your future bundle of joy.

Changes in Mom: One major tell-tale sign of pregnancy is a missed period. You may experience some implantation bleeding, but not true menstrual bleeding. Hormonal changes will occur to support the new pregnancy, and this may come with some PMS-like symptoms.

Foods to Enjoy: Spinach, beets, salmon, avocado, walnut, banana, eggs, and milk or dairy-free milk alternative.

Month 1 Sample Meal Plan

During your first month of pregnancy, you are hopefully feeling just as you were before you were eating for two and symptoms like morning sickness or heartburn have not struck. Take advantage of this time by eating pregnancy-fueling foods that are simple to make and help support this important month of your journey.

	BREAKFAST	LUNCH	DINNER	SNACK/DESSERT
DAY 1	Avocado Egg Salad Toast (page 42)	3 ounces skipjack tuna salad with whole grain crackers, olives, carrot sticks, and 1 apple	Ginger Shrimp Stir-Fry (page 48) with ½ cup brown rice	Roasted Beet Hummus (page 52) with celery sticks
DAY 2	Roasted Granola (page 54) with Greek yogurt and fresh berries	Leftover Ginger Shrimp Stir-Fry with ½ cup brown rice	Pasta with Vegan Avocado Pesto (page 44)	Sliced apple with almond butter
DAY 3	Power-Packed Oats (page 38)	Leftover Pasta with Vegan Avocado Pesto	Almost-Sushi Salmon Bowls (page 49)	Leftover Roasted Beet Hummus with celery sticks
DAY 4	Scrambled eggs with whole grain toast and banana	Leftover Almost-Sushi Salmon Bowl and 1 orange	Chickpea, Beet, and Mango Bowl (page 45)	Hydrating Watermelon Fruit Pop (page 55)
DAY 5	Leftover Roasted Granola with Greek yogurt and fresh berries	Leftover Chickpea, Beet, and Mango Bowl	Chicken Thighs with Parmesan-Covered Charred Broccoli (page 46)	Nori-Wrapped Avocado (page 53)
DAY 6	Avocado Egg Salad Toast (page 42)	Leftover Chicken Thighs with Parmesan-Covered Charred Broccoli	The Balanced Shepherd's Pie (page 50) with green salad	Leftover Hydrating Watermelon Fruit Pop
DAY 7	Brussels Baked Omelet (page 41)	Leftover Balanced Shepherd's Pie and 1 banana	Wild Salmon Salad (page 43)	6 chocolate-dipped strawberries

Certain chemicals like BPA and phthalates can play a negative role in pregnancy outcomes. These chemicals can be found in personal care products, household cleaning items, and in your food packaging.

Now that you are eating for two, make a point to avoid food packaged in BPA-lined containers (like many canned soups), using plastic wrapping on hot food, and microwaving food in plastic containers. When possible, store hot leftovers in glass containers instead of plastic. When heating food in the microwave, place the food on a microwave-safe dish before heating instead of cooking the food in plastic. These small changes can play a positive role in your pregnancy and your future baby's health.

Month 2: Thriving Two-gether

Once you enter your second month of pregnancy, you may notice some changes in your body. You are still very early in your pregnancy, so if you aren't experiencing any symptoms, that's no cause for concern. Some people feel absolutely no symptoms while others experience every ailment under the sun. Experiencing symptoms is not an indication of a healthy pregnancy.

Since you may be experiencing some nausea or morning sickness, focus on foods that may help combat these symptoms. Consuming fresh ginger and foods rich in the nutrient vitamin B_6 may offer some relief. Some B_6-rich foods include tofu, nuts, and chickpeas. At this time, your baby's neural tube is continuing to develop, so key nutrients like folic acid, choline, and vitamin B_{12} continue to be important to support this.

To assist baby's brain development, DHA omega-3 fatty acid intake should be prioritized. This nutrient is found primarily in many fish and seafood options. If mom is able to tolerate it, eating low-mercury seafood two times a week is an excellent way to support baby's brain health. Shrimp, salmon, and scallops are all wonderful choices. If you can't handle these foods, make sure you are supplementing appropriately with a DHA supplement.

Iodine is another brain-promoting nutrient that is needed during pregnancy. Foods like nori seaweed snacks, seafood, and even iodized salt can help you meet your iodine needs.

WHAT TO EXPECT THIS MONTH

How Baby Is Developing: Baby's neural tube continues to develop. Additionally, baby's face is in the beginning stages of development, as well as the start of the formation of vital organs like the liver, kidney, and lungs—although they won't be fully functioning until later in pregnancy. The brain is also developing.

Changes in Mom: Common symptoms include heartburn, nausea/morning sickness, tender breasts, mood swings, exhaustion, food cravings, and smell aversions.

Foods to Enjoy: Shrimp (if able to tolerate), beets, chia seeds, fresh ginger (for nausea relief), tofu, nori (seaweed), whole grain pasta, fresh or frozen fruit (any), and chickpeas.

EXERCISING WITH BABY ON BOARD

Some benefits of exercise during pregnancy include reduced back pain, constipation symptom management, reduced risk of preeclampsia and gestational diabetes, mood support, possible delivery help, and healthy weight management.

According to the American College of Gynecology, pregnant people should aim for at least 150 minutes of moderate-intensity aerobic activity per week. If this value is more than what you were doing pre-pregnancy, you should gradually work up to this goal and make sure your exercise plan is okay with your doctor before you begin.

Month 2 Sample Meal Plan

This month's meal plan takes into account two things: (1) you're eating to support your baby's growth and development, and (2) the sight of anything heavy or the smell of anything strong may put you in a tizzy. This meal plan is balanced and nutrient-dense yet suggests lighter offerings that are easy to tolerate. Vitamin B_6 and ginger-heavy recipes may help some people with nausea relief, too.

	BREAKFAST	LUNCH	DINNER	SNACK/ DESSERT
DAY 1	Ginger-Cauliflower Smoothie (page 36)	Grilled cheese sandwich and sliced fresh tomatoes	Grandma's Homemade Chicken Noodle Soup (page 51)	Nori-Wrapped Avocado (page 53)
DAY 2	Banana-Chia Pudding (page 40)	Leftover Grandma's Homemade Chicken Noodle Soup	Chickpea, Beet, and Mango Bowl (page 45)	Leftover Nori-Wrapped Avocado
DAY 3	Power-Packed Oats (page 38)	Leftover Chickpea, Beet, and Mango Bowl	Ginger Shrimp Stir-Fry (page 48) (swap out shrimp for tofu if shrimp can't be tolerated this month)	Hydrating Watermelon Fruit Pop (page 55)
DAY 4	Ginger-Cauliflower Smoothie (page 36)	Leftover Ginger Shrimp Stir-Fry	Thai-Inspired Green Curry with Chicken (page 47) over ½ cup quinoa	Berries with fresh whipped cream
DAY 5	Leftover Banana-Chia Pudding	Leftover Thai-Inspired Green Curry with Chicken over ½ cup quinoa	Chicken Thighs with Parmesan-Covered Charred Broccoli (page 46)	Air-popped popcorn topped with nutritional yeast
DAY 6	Avocado Egg Salad Toast (page 42)	Leftover Chicken Thighs with Parmesan-Covered Charred Broccoli	Pasta with Vegan Avocado Pesto (page 44)	Leftover Hydrating Watermelon Fruit Pop
DAY 7	Egg white omelet with spinach and pasteurized feta cheese	Leftover Pasta with Vegan Avocado Pesto	Almost-Sushi Salmon Bowls (page 49)	Chocolate-covered frozen banana

Month 3: Nourishing Your Fetus

You are in your final month of your first trimester and are likely getting used to the idea of *being a mom* within the next few months. Your baby is growing and developing and by the end of this month is officially called a fetus.

To combat fatigue that you may be feeling, choose foods that are considered whole grains like quinoa, avocado, and cauliflower. The fiber found in whole grains can help combat any constipation symptoms you may be experiencing as well.

Baby's bones are beginning to harden, and its fingernails are beginning to grow this month. To support baby's bone health, calcium-rich foods like tofu and milk are key to ensure baby is getting what it needs. Additionally, as baby's needs increase, you may need to start bumping up your calorie intake in general.

WHAT TO EXPECT THIS MONTH

How Baby Is Developing: The baby is now called a fetus and many exciting features begin to develop, including buds for future teeth, soft nails, bones and muscles, and intestines.

Changes in Mom: Tender breasts, weight gain, lower back pain, fatigue, food aversions, food cravings, constipation, and morning sickness.

Foods to Enjoy: Mango, strawberry, mushrooms, quinoa, chicken, carrots, avocado, and cauliflower.

Month 3 Sample Meal Plan

Your baby is depending on you to eat nutrient-dense food to supply it with the nutrients it needs to grow and develop. During the third month of pregnancy, natural energy boosters along with bland and easy foods are key to support your nutrition needs this month.

	BREAKFAST	LUNCH	DINNER	SNACK/DESSERT
DAY 1	Nix the Nausea Smoothie (page 37)	Homemade English muffin pizza and 1 plum	Grandma's Homemade Chicken Noodle Soup (page 51)	Roasted Beet Hummus (page 52) with celery sticks
DAY 2	Banana-Chia Pudding (page 40)	Leftover Grandma's Homemade Chicken Noodle Soup	Wild Salmon Salad (page 43)	Nori-Wrapped Avocado (page 53)
DAY 3	Leftover Nix the Nausea Smoothie	Leftover Wild Salmon Salad	Chickpea, Beet, and Mango Bowl (page 45)	Leftover Roasted Beet Hummus with celery sticks
DAY 4	Leftover Banana-Chia Pudding	Leftover Chickpea, Beet, and Mango Bowl	Pasta with Vegan Avocado Pesto (page 44)	Leftover Nori-Wrapped Avocado
DAY 5	Power-Packed Oats (page 38)	Leftover Pasta with Vegan Avocado Pesto	The Balanced Shepherd's Pie (page 50)	Air-popped Parmesan popcorn
DAY 6	Brussels Baked Omelet (page 41)	Leftover Grandma's Homemade Chicken Noodle Soup	Almost-Sushi Salmon Bowls (page 49)	Sliced apple and nut butter
DAY 7	Leftover Power-Packed Oats	Leftover Balanced Shepherd's Pie	Leftover Almost-Sushi Salmon Bowls	Hydrating Watermelon Fruit Pop (page 55)

Immunity Boost Smoothie

DAIRY-FREE, GLUTEN-FREE, VEGETARIAN

SERVES 2

PREP TIME: 5 minutes

This vitamin C–packed smoothie is great during flu season—and for anyone who has tested positive for group B strep or who is trying to avoid premature rupture of membranes or placental abruption.

1 cup frozen pineapple or mango

1 banana

¾ cup unsweetened plain almond milk

½ cup ice

¼ cup 100 percent orange juice

2 tablespoons collagen powder or other pregnancy-safe protein powder

1 tablespoon fresh lemon juice

2 teaspoons pure maple syrup

½ teaspoon ground cinnamon

¼ teaspoon ground ginger

In a blender, blend the pineapple, banana, almond milk, ice, orange juice, collagen powder, lemon juice, maple syrup, cinnamon, and ginger until smooth. Serve immediately or store in the refrigerator for up to 2 days.

Ingredient tip: Adding a few tablespoons of plain whole-milk yogurt or unsweetened almond butter will provide zinc, which fights infection and illness. If your pregnancy diet includes honey, it can be used instead of maple syrup in this recipe.

Per serving: Calories: 168; Total Fat: 1g; Saturated Fat: <1g; Cholesterol: 0mg; Sodium: 68mg; Carbohydrates: 36g; Fiber: 4g; Protein: 7g

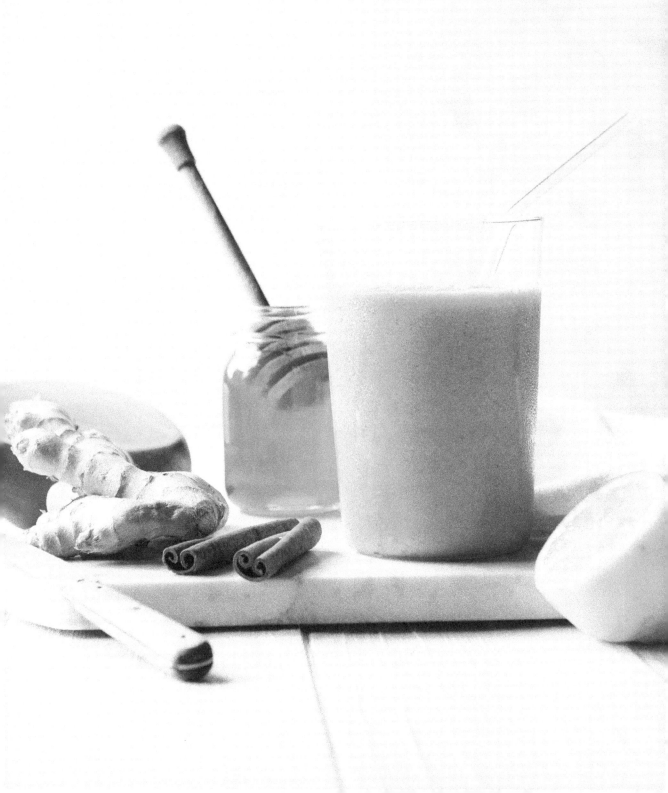

Ginger-Cauliflower Smoothie

GLUTEN-FREE, NUT-FREE, VEGETARIAN

SERVES 1

PREP TIME: 5 minutes / **COOK TIME:** 5 minutes

This smoothie is an excellent solution if you're experiencing nausea and having a difficult time getting in fruits and veggies. The fresh ginger offers some potential nausea relief, while the variety of fruits and veggies gives this smoothie a boost of nutrition. The addition of Greek yogurt provides some fat and protein to help you feel satisfied all morning long.

½ cup packaged frozen riced cauliflower

1 cup frozen strawberries

½ banana, sliced

½ cup cubed frozen mango

½ cup vanilla reduced-fat Greek yogurt

½ cup ice

½-inch piece ginger, chopped, or
  ½ teaspoon ground ginger

1. Microwave the riced cauliflower according to the package directions. Set aside and cool in the refrigerator.

2. In a blender, blend the cauliflower, strawberries, banana, mango, yogurt, ice, and ginger until smooth. Serve immediately or store in the refrigerator for up to 2 days.

Substitution tip: Coconut, almond, soy, or oat milk yogurt can be substituted for the Greek yogurt to make this smoothie vegan-friendly.

Per serving: Calories: 287; Total Fat: 3g; Saturated Fat: 1g; Cholesterol: 11mg; Sodium: 66mg; Carbohydrates: 57g; Fiber: 10g; Protein: 13g

Nix the Nausea Smoothie

VEGETARIAN

SERVES 2

PREP TIME: 5 minutes

If you haven't experienced first-trimester nausea yet, you are a blessed being. For the majority of you with queasy stomachs announcing themselves at any time of day, keep these ingredients stocked so you can get in at least a little sustenance.

1 cup full-fat coconut milk

1 cup cooked rolled oats

1 cup frozen strawberries

1 banana

½ cup ice

½ cup plain whole-milk yogurt or kefir

2 tablespoons collagen peptides (or other pregnancy-safe protein powder)

1 or 2 dried ginger capsules

1. In a blender, blend the coconut milk, oats, strawberries, banana, ice, yogurt, and collagen.

2. Open the ginger capsule and empty the contents into the blender, discarding the capsule. Blend until smooth.

3. Serve immediately or store in the refrigerator for up to 2 days.

Substitution tip: To make this smoothie dairy-free, swap the yogurt for a plant-based one. To make it vegetarian, choose a plant-based protein powder instead of collagen peptides. Both yogurt and kefir are probiotic dairy beverages that can be used in many recipes interchangeably. They are made differently and thus end up containing different strains of beneficial bacteria, but both typically taste tart. Kefir typically has more fat than yogurt, but it also has more protein and probiotics.

Per serving: Calories: 502; Total Fat: 28g; Saturated Fat: 22g; Cholesterol: 15mg; Sodium: 154mg; Carbohydrates: 48g; Fiber: 6g; Protein: 24g

Power-Packed Oats

DAIRY-FREE, GLUTEN-FREE, VEGETARIAN

SERVES 2

PREP TIME: 2 minutes / **COOK TIME:** 5 minutes

While oats have a well-balanced nutritional profile for a grain, I know most of you pregnant mamas are always trying to get in more protein, so I added eggs. Oats are the perfect bland breakfast base for anyone struggling with traditional morning sickness. If you're feeling up for it, I've included optional toppings to amp up the antioxidants, omega-3s, and probiotics.

1 cup rolled oats

2 cups almond milk (substitute filtered water for nut-free)

2 large eggs, lightly beaten

Pinch salt

Few drops pure vanilla extract (optional)

Cherries, pitted, for topping (optional)

Apricots, pitted, for topping (optional)

Chia seeds, for topping (optional)

Plain whole-milk yogurt, for topping (optional, if not dairy-free)

1. In a medium saucepan over medium-high heat, stir together the oats, almond milk, eggs, salt, and vanilla (if using) and bring to a boil.

2. Reduce the heat to low and simmer for 5 minutes, or until the liquid is absorbed, stirring occasionally to fully incorporate the egg.

3. Serve warm, topped with cherries, apricots, chia seeds, and yogurt (if using).

Ingredient tip: If you're having a hard time stomaching eggs, add a scoop or two of collagen powder to your finished oatmeal instead.

Per serving: Calories: 316; Total Fat: 15g; Saturated Fat: 2g; Cholesterol: 200mg; Sodium: 441mg; Carbohydrates: 30g; Fiber: 7g; Protein: 14g

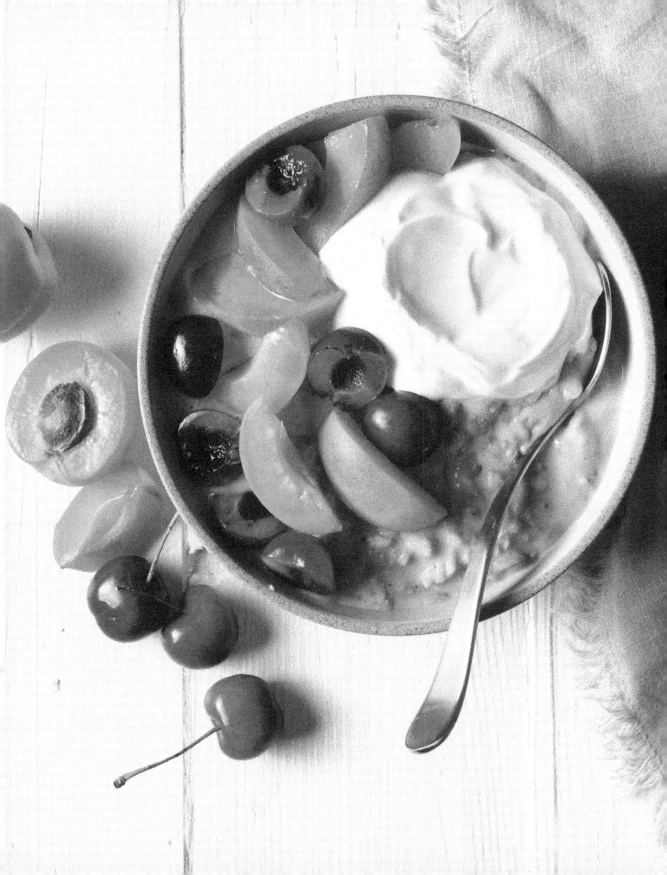

Banana-Chia Pudding

DAIRY-FREE, GLUTEN-FREE, VEGETARIAN

SERVES 4

PREP TIME: 10 minutes, plus 6 hours to chill

Chia pudding is great for busy mornings when you don't have time to cook a full break-fast. This is a much more nutritious choice than grabbing a donut on the way out the door. Mixing fiber-rich chia seeds with liquid and allowing the combination to sit overnight creates a gel-like consistency that is very close to classic pudding.

2 large ripe bananas, mashed

2 cups plain unsweetened almond milk

6 tablespoons chia seeds

1 tablespoon pure maple syrup

1 teaspoon ground cinnamon

1. In a medium bowl, combine the bananas, almond milk, chia seeds, maple syrup, and cinnamon and mix together.

2. Set aside for 30 minutes, then stir again.

3. Cover and refrigerate for 6 hours or overnight before serving.

Substitution tip: Use coconut milk instead of almond milk to make this breakfast taste similar to a coconut–banana cream pie! Top with slivered almonds for an extra protein boost.

Per serving: Calories: 183; Total Fat: 7g; Saturated Fat: <1g; Cholesterol: 0mg; Sodium: 88mg; Carbohydrates: 28g; Fiber: 10g; Protein: 4g

Brussels Baked Omelet

DAIRY-FREE, GLUTEN-FREE, NUT-FREE, VEGETARIAN

SERVES 4

PREP TIME: 10 minutes / **COOK TIME:** 20 minutes

Mom and baby get a lot of good things from this simple egg bake, which is full of flavor from ingredients that contain nutrients deeply needed during the third month of pregnancy. Brussels sprouts are brimming with folate, magnesium, vitamin C, vitamin A, and choline.

8 large eggs

1 teaspoon dried basil

½ teaspoon dried thyme

½ teaspoon salt

2 cups diced Brussels sprouts

½ cup diced red onion

1. Preheat the oven to 325°F. Line a 9-by-9-inch pan with parchment paper.

2. In a large bowl, whisk the eggs until blended, then slowly whisk in the basil, thyme, and salt.

3. Pour the egg mixture into the parchment paper–lined pan. Sprinkle the Brussels sprouts and onion on top of the eggs.

4. Bake for 15 minutes, or until it begins to puff and turn slightly golden. Let cool for 5 minutes before cutting into squares for serving.

Ingredient tip: If you can nab some fresh basil or thyme for this dish, do it! They taste better and have greater antioxidant potential than dried herbs. The general rule of thumb when converting recipes with fresh herbs is to triple the measurement of the dried.

Per serving: Calories: 171; Total Fat: 11g; Saturated Fat: 3g; Cholesterol: 326mg; Sodium: 450mg; Carbohydrates: 6g; Fiber: 2g; Protein: 12g

Avocado Egg Salad Toast

NUT-FREE, VEGETARIAN

SERVES 2

PREP TIME: 10 minutes

This recipe can help those trying to hit their egg quota (but are tired of eating them baked, fried, and scrambled). Eggs really are a magical pregnancy food, as they help you nail a hard-to-meet nutrient requirement: choline. This recipe's nutrient profile boasts other greats as well: vitamin A, folate, vitamin B$_{12}$, iodine, magnesium, and zinc.

4 hard-boiled eggs, peeled and chopped

1 medium avocado, pitted and peeled

2 tablespoons plain whole-milk yogurt

1 tablespoon fresh lemon juice

1 tablespoon minced shallots

1 teaspoon Dijon mustard

2 sourdough toast slices

2 cooked nitrate- and nitrite-free bacon slices, crumbled (optional)

1. In a medium bowl, mash together the eggs, avocado, yogurt, lemon juice, shallots, and mustard.

2. Spread the egg salad onto the two toast slices. Garnish with bacon (if using).

Ingredient tip: You can easily make this recipe gluten-free by using gluten-free bread or a lettuce wrap in lieu of the sourdough. Please note that common allergen consumption during pregnancy has been shown to help with future tolerance in baby, so if you can eat it without physical side effects, don't feel guilty about enjoying real bread here and there.

Per serving: Calories: 368; Total Fat: 23g; Saturated Fat: 5g; Cholesterol: 328mg; Sodium: 356mg; Carbohydrates: 26g; Fiber: 7g; Protein: 17g

Wild Salmon Salad

DAIRY-FREE, GLUTEN-FREE, NUT-FREE

SERVES 2

PREP TIME: 5 minutes

I adore this salad for its winning combination of tasty ingredients that each bring something needed to the first-trimester nutrient equation. Magnesium, iodine, omega-3s, choline, folate, and vitamins A, B$_{12}$, and C are all covered in this dish. If you have an aversion to fish, consider trying it cold! Oftentimes the lowered temperature can change everything.

¼ cup extra-virgin olive oil

¼ cup red wine vinegar

1 tablespoon fresh lime juice

½ teaspoon garlic powder

½ teaspoon chili powder

½ teaspoon salt

4 cups arugula

1 cup cooked or canned salmon, flaked
  with a fork

½ orange, peeled and chopped

½ bell pepper, any color, diced

½ cucumber, diced

½ cup cooked quinoa

¼ cup sunflower seeds

¼ cup minced fresh cilantro

1. In a small bowl, make the dressing by whisking together the olive oil, red wine vinegar, lime juice, garlic powder, chili powder, and salt.

2. In a large bowl, combine the arugula, salmon, orange, bell pepper, cucumber, quinoa, sunflower seeds, and cilantro and toss to combine. Add the dressing and toss again until combined.

3. Divide between two plates and serve.

Ingredient tip: This recipe is ideal for leftover cooked salmon, but one cup of salmon is about equal to a 6-ounce can of wild-caught salmon.

Per serving: Calories: 483; Total Fat: 35g; Saturated Fat: 5g; Cholesterol: 37mg; Sodium: 455mg; Carbohydrates: 25g; Fiber: 5g; Protein: 22g

Pasta with Vegan Avocado Pesto

DAIRY-FREE, VEGETARIAN

SERVES 4

PREP TIME: 5 minutes

This pesto recipe takes advantage of the natural creaminess of avocado to make a rich sauce that is pregnancy-fueling and chock-full of healthy fats and important nutrients like folate. This is a great recipe to make on a busy weeknight when you need dinner on the table quickly.

1 large ripe avocado, pitted and peeled

½ cup fresh basil leaves

½ cup fresh baby arugula

½ cup pine nuts

½ cup walnut pieces

¼ cup extra-virgin olive oil

1 tablespoon jarred minced garlic

Juice of 1 lemon

½ teaspoon salt

¼ teaspoon freshly ground black pepper

2 cups cooked whole grain
   spaghetti, drained

1. In a food processor, blend the avocado, basil, arugula, pine nuts, walnuts, olive oil, garlic, lemon juice, salt, and pepper. Puree until smooth, scraping down the sides as you go.

2. Toss sauce with the pasta and serve.

Ingredient tip: The pesto can be used as a sandwich condiment, a vegetable dip, and a sauce for white fish. Try topping this dish with grilled shrimp or scallops.

Per serving: Calories: 517; Total Fat: 42g; Saturated Fat: 6g; Cholesterol: 0mg; Sodium: 316mg; Carbohydrates: 33g; Fiber: 10g; Protein: 10g

Chickpea, Beet, and Mango Bowl

DAIRY-FREE, GLUTEN-FREE, VEGETARIAN

SERVES 4

PREP TIME: 10 minutes / **COOK TIME:** 35 minutes

This easy-prep dish is a wonderful pregnancy-fueling dinner. Natural folate from the beets is paired with plant-based protein and fiber from the quinoa and chickpeas to create a satisfying and nourishing dinner that tastes great as a leftover dish, too.

8 ounces beets, peeled and cubed

2 tablespoons extra-virgin olive oil, divided

1 (15-ounce) can chickpeas, drained, rinsed, and dried

1 tablespoon Italian seasoning

4 tablespoons jarred pesto or Vegan Avocado Pesto (page 44)

4 tablespoons red wine vinegar

2 cups cooked quinoa

2 avocados, pitted, peeled, and sliced

1 mango, peeled, cored, and chopped

1. Preheat the oven to 425°F.

2. On a baking sheet, toss the beets with 1 tablespoon of olive oil.

3. Toss the chickpeas with the remaining tablespoon of olive oil and the Italian seasoning and place them on the other side of the baking sheet. Bake for 20 minutes until the beets are tender.

4. In a small bowl, whisk the pesto with the red wine vinegar.

5. Place a ½ cup of quinoa in each bowl, covering the bottom. Add the chickpeas, beets, avocado, and mango in sections. Drizzle with the pesto.

Substitution tip: Frozen mangos that have been defrosted can be substituted for fresh mango. Any ancient grain can be used in place of quinoa for an equally satisfying dish. Try this recipe using spelt, sorghum, or even brown rice if quinoa is not available.

Per serving: Calories: 522; Total Fat: 27g; Saturated Fat: 4g; Cholesterol: 0mg; Sodium: 295mg; Carbohydrates: 61g; Fiber: 15g; Protein: 13g

Chicken Thighs with Parmesan-Covered Charred Broccoli

GLUTEN-FREE, NUT-FREE

SERVES 4

PREP TIME: 5 minutes / **COOK TIME:** 30 minutes

Chicken thighs are a budget-friendly protein choice that can cook up juicy with little effort. I keep the skin on, as it contains a greater concentration of fat-soluble vitamins like the active form of vitamin A. This one-skillet wonder also includes broccoli, which contains several month-two nutrients (like vitamin C, choline, and folate), and Parmesan, which is rich in several B vitamins, vitamin A, calcium, and zinc.

3 tablespoons ghee or butter, melted and divided

6 bone-in, skin-on chicken thighs (about 1½ pounds total)

½ teaspoon salt, plus more for seasoning

Freshly ground black pepper

3 garlic cloves, minced

1 large broccoli head, chopped

½ cup grated Parmesan cheese

1. Preheat the oven to 425°F.

2. In a cast-iron skillet, melt 1 tablespoon of ghee over medium-high heat. Season the chicken thighs lightly on all sides with salt and pepper and carefully place them into the hot skillet, skin-side down, and cook for 10 minutes. Sprinkle the garlic around the chicken and cook for another 5 minutes.

3. Meanwhile, in a large bowl, toss the broccoli in the remaining 2 tablespoons of ghee and ½ teaspoon of salt.

4. Turn the chicken thighs over and scatter the broccoli evenly over the top of the chicken.

5. Place the skillet into the oven and roast for 15 minutes, until the internal temperature of the chicken has reached 165°F and the broccoli has begun to char on top.

6. Immediately sprinkle the Parmesan over the broccoli so it melts before serving. Place 1 to 2 pieces of chicken and some of the cheese-covered broccoli onto each plate and serve.

Per serving: Calories: 531; Total Fat: 42g; Saturated Fat: 19g; Cholesterol: 183mg; Sodium: 309mg; Carbohydrates: 9g; Fiber: 3g; Protein: 33g

DAIRY-FREE, GLUTEN-FREE

SERVES 6

PREP TIME: 10 minutes / **COOK TIME:** 20 minutes

The spices in curry beautifully aid digestion, which can start to feel funky early on in pregnancy, while the bone broth and coconut milk soothe an unsettled tummy. If you prefer a thicker curry, reduce the amount of broth. Curry is often served over white rice, but don't let that limit you. Try zucchini noodles or quinoa, or eat it plain like stew or soup. If using store-bought broth, be aware of the potentially higher sodium content and consider not adding any more salt.

1 tablespoon coconut oil

1 medium yellow onion, diced

2 garlic cloves, minced

½ teaspoon dried ginger

½ teaspoon salt

1½ pounds boneless, skin-on chicken
 breast, cut into ½-inch pieces

3 cups green beans, trimmed and cut into
 1-inch pieces

2 sweet potatoes, cut into 1-inch cubes

1 (13.5-ounce) can full-fat coconut milk

2 cups Slow Cooker Beef Bone Broth
 (page 87) or store-bought

4 tablespoons green curry paste

2 teaspoons fish sauce

Juice of 1 lime

1. In a medium pot, warm the coconut oil over medium-high heat. Add the onion, garlic, ginger, and salt, stir to combine, and cook for 5 minutes.

2. Add the chicken, green beans, and sweet potatoes and cook for another 5 minutes, until the chicken is cooked through.

3. Stir in the coconut milk, broth, curry paste, fish sauce, and lime juice. Bring to a simmer and cook until the sweet potatoes are tender, about 10 minutes.

Ingredient tip: Leaving the skin on the chicken will add both flavor and nutrients (hello, collagen!).

Per serving: Calories: 447; Total Fat: 28g; Saturated Fat: 17g; Cholesterol: 15mg; Sodium: 862mg; Carbohydrates: 23g; Fiber: 5g; Protein: 30g

Ginger Shrimp Stir-Fry

DAIRY-FREE, NUT-FREE

SERVES 4

PREP TIME: 10 minutes / **COOK TIME:** 15 minutes

Fresh ginger can be a welcome addition to an early pregnancy diet for natural nausea relief. Combining ginger with shrimp may help get some seafood into your diet and help ingest the important fatty acid DHA. If you simply cannot stomach shrimp, tofu is a nice substitute.

½ cup vegetable broth

¼ cup fresh lemon juice

2 tablespoons low-sodium soy sauce

3 garlic cloves, minced

1 tablespoon grated fresh ginger

2 teaspoons sesame oil

1 red bell pepper, sliced

1 cup broccoli florets

1 cup sliced button mushrooms

½ yellow onion, sliced

½ cup fresh sugar snap peas

1 tablespoon thinly sliced fresh ginger

1 pound shrimp, peeled and deveined

1 (10-ounce) bag frozen cauliflower rice, cooked according to package directions

1. In a medium bowl, whisk the vegetable broth, lemon juice, soy sauce, garlic, and ginger.

2. In a large skillet, heat the sesame oil over medium-high heat. Cook the bell pepper, broccoli, mushrooms, onions, snap peas, and ginger for 5 minutes, or until the onions are softened. Set the vegetable mixture aside.

3. In the same skillet, cook the shrimp until pink, about 3 minutes. Add the vegetables and sauce to the skillet and cook for 2 minutes until hot. Serve over cauliflower rice.

Substitution tip: Swap out the shrimp for firm tofu to make this meal a vegan-friendly dish that gives a boost of calcium and plant-based protein.

Per serving: Calories: 156; Total Fat: 3g; Saturated Fat: <1g; Cholesterol: 120mg; Sodium: 675mg; Carbohydrates: 13g; Fiber: 4g; Protein: 23g

Almost-Sushi Salmon Bowls

DAIRY-FREE, GLUTEN-FREE

SERVES 4

PREP TIME: 10 minutes / **COOK TIME:** 10 minutes

If you're completely avoiding raw fish but still craving your favorite Japanese restaurant, this bowl is perfect for you. Salmon is full of brain-building omega-3s that support your baby's development, as well as your postpartum mental health.

1 tablespoon coconut oil

1 pound salmon fillet, cut into chunks

½ teaspoon salt

4 cups cooked brown rice

1 medium cucumber, diced

1 medium avocado, pitted, peeled, and sliced

½ cup shredded carrot

4 nori sheets, cut into strips

2 scallions, both white and green parts, sliced

3 tablespoons sesame seeds

2 limes, halved

1. In a medium skillet, heat the coconut oil over medium-high heat.

2. Season the salmon all over with the salt and cook until opaque, 2 to 3 minutes per side. Remove from the heat and set aside.

3. Divide the rice among four bowls and top with the salmon. Sprinkle the cucumber, avocado, carrot, nori, scallions, and sesame seeds over the salmon. Squeeze the limes over each portion before serving.

Cooking tip: To make this dish seem even more like sushi, refrigerate before serving. Plus, cold foods tend to trigger nausea less than warm or hot foods. Win-win!

Per serving: Calories: 381; Total Fat: 18g; Saturated Fat: 5g; Cholesterol: 84mg; Sodium: 312mg; Carbohydrates: 26g; Fiber: 6g; Protein: 28g

The Balanced Shepherd's Pie

GLUTEN-FREE, NUT-FREE, FREEZER-FRIENDLY

SERVES 4

PREP TIME: 10 minutes / **COOK TIME:** 30 minutes

Traditional shepherd's pie is very high in carbohydrates from the mashed potato topping. This more nutritionally balanced version uses mashed cauliflower. You can also swap out the cauliflower for a root vegetable like sweet potato or celery root.

3 tablespoons ghee or grass-fed butter, divided

4½ cups chopped cauliflower florets

¼ teaspoon garlic powder

¾ teaspoon salt, divided

1 cup packed minced fresh spinach

2 medium carrots, peeled and diced

1 small yellow onion, diced

2 garlic cloves, minced

1 pound ground turkey

1 (15-ounce) can diced tomatoes, drained

2 tablespoons tomato paste

2 tablespoons coconut aminos

1 teaspoon dried thyme

½ teaspoon freshly ground black pepper

1. Preheat the oven to 400°F. Grease all sides of a 9-inch square casserole dish using 1 tablespoon of ghee.

2. In a large skillet, melt 1 tablespoon of ghee over medium-high heat. Add the cauliflower, garlic powder, and ¼ teaspoon of salt. Cook until tender, about 10 minutes.

3. In another skillet, melt the remaining tablespoon of ghee over medium-high heat. Add the spinach, carrots, onion, garlic, and remaining ½ teaspoon of salt and cook for 5 minutes, stirring continually. Add the turkey and continue to cook for about 10 minutes, breaking the turkey up as it cooks and stirring occasionally, until the meat is cooked through. Add the diced tomatoes, tomato paste, coconut aminos, thyme, and pepper and stir to combine. Remove from the heat.

4. Transfer the cauliflower from the skillet to a food processor and blend until smooth.

5. Spoon the turkey mixture into the casserole dish and spread out evenly. Spoon the cauliflower mash over the turkey and spread evenly. Bake for 15 minutes, until the cauliflower starts to brown on top.

Per serving: Calories: 297; Total Fat: 12g; Saturated Fat: 6g; Cholesterol: 76mg; Sodium: 571mg; Carbohydrates: 18g; Fiber: 6g; Protein: 31g

Grandma's Homemade Chicken Noodle Soup

DAIRY-FREE, NUT-FREE, FREEZER-FRIENDLY

SERVES 6

PREP TIME: 5 minutes / **COOK TIME:** 1½ hours

....

Chicken noodle soup is normally well-tolerated during the first trimester and is chock-full of important nutrients. Not only is it nourishing, but it can help keep you hydrated, which can be challenging if you're struggling with nausea.

....

1 (2-pound) whole chicken, cut into 8 pieces

8 cups cold water

1 yellow onion, diced

3 carrots, peeled and diced

2 celery stalks, diced

2 dill sprigs

1 cup fine egg noodles

1 cup sliced button mushrooms

1 cup shredded fresh spinach

½ teaspoon salt

½ teaspoon freshly ground black pepper

1. Place the chicken in a large pot. Pour in the water and bring to a boil. Skim off the fat.

2. Add the onion, carrot, celery, and dill. Cover and simmer for 1½ hours.

3. Strain off the fat, remove the chicken and carrots from the soup, and let cool.

4. Add the noodles and mushrooms and cook for about 8 minutes until tender.

5. Cut the chicken and carrots into bite-size pieces and add them back to the soup. Discard the chicken bones and skin. Add the spinach, salt, and pepper and cook covered, until the spinach is wilted.

Time-saving tip: Double this recipe and freeze portions of this soup for busy nights when nothing will do except for some homemade chicken noodle soup.

....

Per serving: Calories: 371; Total Fat: 13g; Saturated Fat: 3g; Cholesterol: 156mg; Sodium: 375mg; Carbohydrates: 12g; Fiber: 2g; Protein: 50g

Roasted Beet Hummus

SERVES 4

DAIRY-FREE, GLUTEN-FREE, NUT-FREE, VEGETARIAN

PREP TIME: 5 minutes

....

Beets are a unique source of betaine, a nutrient made from choline. Betaine has been touted for lowering inflammation, which is crucial for placental health. Increased betaine intake during pregnancy has also been linked to better infant cognitive development, so bring on the beets!

....

2 medium beets, roasted

1 (15-ounce) can chickpeas, rinsed
  and drained

¼ cup tahini

¼ cup extra-virgin olive oil

1 tablespoon fresh lemon juice

2 teaspoons coconut aminos

½ teaspoon ground ginger

½ teaspoon garlic powder

½ teaspoon salt

1. In a food processor, blend the beets, chickpeas, tahini, olive oil, lemon juice, coconut aminos, ginger, garlic powder, and salt, scraping down the sides with a silicone spatula, until smooth.

2. Place in an airtight container and refrigerate for 1 hour before serving for a firmer consistency.

3. The hummus can be stored in the refrigerator for up to 5 days.

Ingredient tip: Coconut aminos, a wheat-free and soy-free alternative to soy sauce, is available in most grocery stores, even Trader Joe's. My husband can't tell the difference—it's that good! Trimmed beets can be scrubbed and roasted in a 400°F oven until easily pierced with a paring knife, about 1 hour. Peel the beets after roasting.

....

Per serving: Calories: 370; Total Fat: 23g; Saturated Fat: 3g; Cholesterol: 0mg; Sodium: 318mg; Carbohydrates: 34g; Fiber: 9g; Protein: 11g

Nori-Wrapped Avocado

DAIRY-FREE, GLUTEN-FREE, NUT-FREE, VEGETARIAN

SERVES 4

PREP TIME: 10 minutes

Iodine is an important nutrient to support baby's brain health, and the need for it increases substantially during pregnancy. One great source of this nutrient is nori seaweed. Pairing nori sheets with folate- and fiber-rich avocado and choline- and vitamin B_{12}-rich egg makes this recipe an ultimate pregnancy-fueling snack that can be enjoyed throughout your entire pregnancy and beyond.

4 ripe avocados, pitted, peeled, and diced

4 hard-boiled eggs, peeled and diced

2 dill sprigs, chopped

⅛ teaspoon salt

Freshly ground black pepper

4 nori sheets

1. In a medium bowl, combine the avocado, egg, and dill. Season with salt and pepper and mix until creamy.

2. Divide the mixture among four sheets of nori and spread evenly. Roll the nori sheet with the mixture inside to form a hand-roll-like snack.

3. Serve immediately and store leftovers in an airtight container in the refrigerator for up to 1 day.

Ingredient tip: Sprinkle these snacks with sesame seeds for an additional boost of healthy fats.

Per serving: Calories: 298; Total Fat: 26g; Saturated Fat: 4g; Cholesterol: 164mg; Sodium: 120mg; Carbohydrates: 13g; Fiber: 10g; Protein: 9g

Roasted Granola

DAIRY-FREE, VEGETARIAN

SERVES 6

PREP TIME: 10 minutes / **COOK TIME:** 45 minutes

Make this granola your go-to when you're craving a sweet and crunchy carb for breakfast and you don't want to eat processed boxed cereal. The cacao added here has a surprising amount of magnesium. And I love the use of oats as a complex breakfast carb, especially when balanced out by the fat in the coconut and seeds.

1 banana

3 tablespoons coconut oil, melted

1 tablespoon unsweetened
   cocoa powder

½ teaspoon ground ginger

½ teaspoon salt

½ teaspoon pure vanilla extract or vanilla
   bean powder

2 cups rolled oats

¼ cup unsweetened coconut flakes

¼ cup pumpkin seeds or sunflower seeds

¼ cup diced dried apricots

1. Preheat the oven to 325°F. Line a baking sheet with parchment paper.

2. In a large mixing bowl, mash the banana with a fork. Whisk in the coconut oil, cocoa powder, ginger, salt, and vanilla until smooth.

3. Add the oats, coconut, and seeds and stir until well coated.

4. Spread the granola onto the prepared baking sheet and bake for 35 to 45 minutes, stirring every 10 minutes, until the granola is dry and golden brown.

5. Allow the granola to cool for 5 minutes, then stir in the dried apricots. Let cool completely on the baking sheet before transferring to an airtight container. The granola can be stored at room temperature for up to 1 week.

Cooking tip: After baking, the granola will be in chunks and clusters, which you can break up by hand. Just be sure to cook it long enough for the moisture to evaporate, which will allow the pieces to break off more easily.

Per serving: Calories: 259; Total Fat: 18g; Saturated Fat: 12g; Cholesterol: 0mg; Sodium: 160mg; Carbohydrates: 23g; Fiber: 5g; Protein: 5g

Hydrating Watermelon Fruit Pop

DAIRY-FREE, GLUTEN-FREE, NUT-FREE, VEGETARIAN, FREEZER-FRIENDLY

SERVES 4

PREP TIME: 5 minutes, plus 6 hours to chill

Staying hydrated is one of the most important things a pregnant mom can do during her pregnancy to help keep herself safe and healthy. While drinking adequate amounts of water is highly recommended, enjoying a frozen fruit pop once in a while can satisfy your sweet tooth and support your hydration at the same time: win-win! Because watermelon is over 90 percent water, this is a logical fruit to use as the focus of these pops.

3 cups chopped watermelon

2 tablespoons granulated sugar

Juice of ½ lime

1. In a blender, blend the watermelon, sugar, and lime juice and process until pureed.

2. Pour into four ice pop molds and freeze for 6 hours or overnight.

Ingredient tip: Add ½ teaspoon of salt to the mixture before serving if you enjoy your watermelon salted. Feel free to get creative with these pops: add a chocolate drizzle for a more decadent treat.

Per serving: Calories: 49; Total Fat: <1g; Saturated Fat: 0g; Cholesterol: 0mg; Sodium: 1mg; Carbohydrates: 13g; Fiber: <1g; Protein: 1g

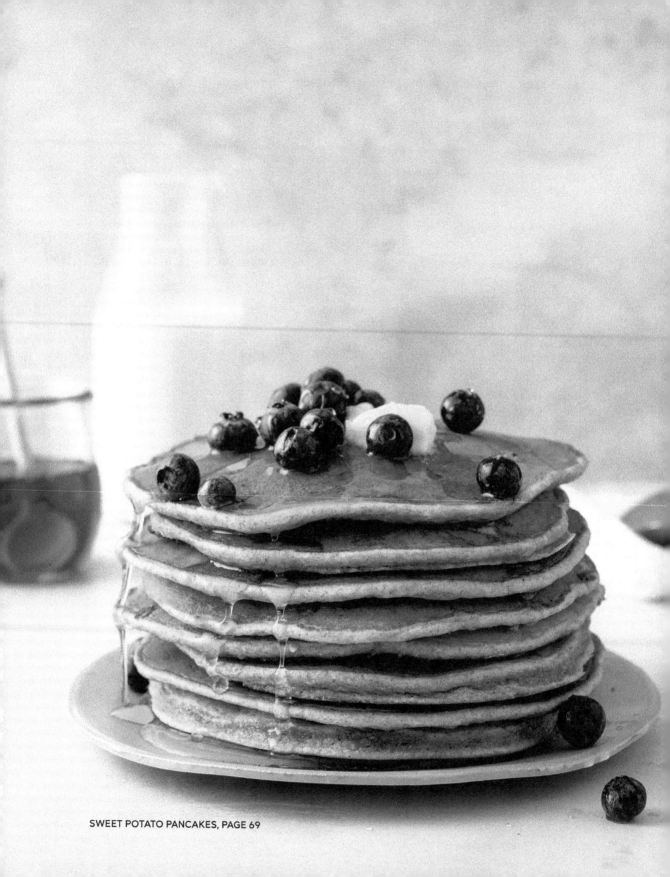

SWEET POTATO PANCAKES, PAGE 69

The Second Trimester

Congratulations on entering your second trimester—the months in which more fetal development occurs and, thankfully, many unwelcome pregnancy symptoms subside. Your belly will likely start popping during this time, if it hasn't already, so it may be time to invest in some maternity clothes. Eating during your second trimester is often an easier task than when you were navigating nausea or fatigue during your first trimester. You may actually feel your best during these months and take advantage of this by eating as many nutrient-rich foods as you can. These types of foods continue to be a priority as you progress in your pregnancy. Enjoy your second trimester, mama!

Month 4: Starting the Second Trimester

Both mom and baby are going through changes in their respective bodies and are progressing in the journey. Eating the right foods will support the natural development and possibly help offer relief to some unwanted side effects, like constipation.

Dairy foods are key this month for a few reasons. For one, milk may relieve heartburn symptoms. Second, baby's bones and teeth require calcium for development. If you aren't taking in enough calcium, the pregnancy will prioritize the baby's needs—meaning you may not have enough calcium to meet your own needs and run the risk of putting your own bone health at risk.

Fiber-rich foods like mushrooms, apples with the skin still on, and whole grains like quinoa can offer some constipation relief. Just make sure to drink enough water, too, as dehydration can also cause constipation.

Protein sources such as eggs and peanut butter are an excellent food for mom to eat. Bonus? Eggs provide important nutrients to support baby's brain development. And although peanut and egg allergies are common, eating these foods during pregnancy does not increase baby's risk of developing these food allergies.

Magnesium is another important mineral to consume for baby's bone support. Sweet potatoes provide natural magnesium and can also satisfy a sweet tooth.

Iodine is a nutrient found in foods like fish, milk, and eggs. Make sure to get in enough of this important nutrient to support baby's brain health. Focusing on this nutrient now can potentially play a large and positive role in baby's brain health throughout its lifetime.

While you may experience headaches for a variety of reasons, including hormone changes, nutrition may offer some relief. Some people also find relief when they limit salt in their diet as well and flavor their food instead with garlic and fresh herbs. It's also important to make sure you're eating enough to avoid headaches. Generally speaking, pregnant people should use the following tips as a guide for what to eat per day:

- 2 or 3 servings of lean protein, or at least 75 grams

- 3 or more servings of whole grains

- 4 or 5 servings of fruits and vegetables (more veggies than fruit preferably)

- 4 servings of calcium-rich food such as dairy and tofu

- At least 1 serving of healthy fat like nuts

Your caloric needs may increase to an extra 340 calories per day during this trimester. This value may vary depending on your pre-pregnancy weight, health status, whether you are pregnant with multiples, and other factors.

WHAT TO EXPECT THIS MONTH

How Baby Is Developing: Baby is starting to hear sound and its kidneys are beginning to function. Your baby's heartbeat may now be audible through a doppler. Eyelids, eyebrows, eyelashes, nails, and hair are formed, and teeth and bones become thicker.

Changes in Mom: Mom may experience round ligament pain (ligaments are literally stretching and growing to support the growing belly and may be felt as stomach pain). Mom may also experience sleeping challenges, bleeding gums, headaches, stuffy nose, constipation, and heartburn.

Foods to Enjoy This Month: Milk, sweet potato, cooked mushrooms, eggs, apples (with skin), peanut butter, whole grains, and water.

Month 4 Sample Meal Plan

Now that the first trimester nausea has hopefully subsided, your diet calls for more variety. Protein-rich and nutrient-dense food are the stars of this sample menu. Food choices are rich in important nutrients that both mom and baby need to develop and grow in a healthy way.

	BREAKFAST	LUNCH	DINNER	SNACK/DESSERT
DAY 1	Sweet Potato Pancakes (page 69) topped with nut butter, 1 teaspoon maple syrup, blueberries	Grilled cheese on whole grain bread with sliced tomato and a pear	Blended Mushroom Burger with Oven-Baked Green Bean Fries (page 79)	1 cup grapes and cheddar cheese cubes
DAY 2	Leftover Sweet Potato Pancakes topped with nut butter, 1 teaspoon maple syrup, blueberries	Leftover Blended Mushroom Burger with Oven-Baked Green Bean Fries	Salmon, Broccoli, and Sweet Potato Sheet Pan (page 85)	Peanut Butter Fruit Dip with Sliced Apples (page 92)
DAY 3	Egg Muffin Cup (page 70) and 1 cup berries	Leftover Salmon, Broccoli, and Sweet Potato Sheet Pan	Nutrient-Dense Bolognese (page 86) over whole grain pasta	Chocolate-Avocado Mousse (page 95)
DAY 4	Leftover Egg Muffin Cup and 1 cup berries	Leftover Nutrient-Dense Bolognese over whole grain pasta	Mediterranean-Inspired Stuffed Sweet Potatoes (page 78)	Leftover Peanut Butter Fruit Dip with Sliced Apples
DAY 5	Whipped Cottage Cheese Berry Bowl (page 68)	Leftover Mediterranean-Inspired Stuffed Sweet Potatoes	Creamy Coconut-Lentil Dal (page 80) with ½ cup brown rice	Ranch Zucchini Chips (page 93)
DAY 6	Leftover Egg Muffin Cup, 1 orange, and 1 slice whole grain toast	Leftover Creamy Coconut-Lentil Dal with ½ cup brown rice	Herbed Lamb with Cauliflower Mash (page 88)	Leftover Ranch Zucchini Chips
DAY 7	Whipped Cottage Cheese Berry Bowl (page 68)	Leftover Herbed Lamb with Cauliflower Mash	Triple Green Pesto Pasta (page 77)	Baked corn chips and salsa with ½ small sliced avocado and black olives

During this month, you are likely to have an anatomy scan. If your health care provider is drawing labs, consider requesting a vitamin D check at this time. Vitamin D plays a positive role in pregnancy outcomes, and a deficiency is quite common, especially during winter months because vitamin D is converted through the skin when exposed to UV light.

If a deficiency is discovered, foods like salmon, eggs, and dairy all contain this nutrient. Other foods, like fortified orange juice, contain vitamin D as well. If supplementation is indicated, don't overdo it—follow the guidance of your health care provider to avoid taking too much. Most health care professionals prefer the vitamin D_3 form of supplementation, as opposed to the vitamin D_2 form, but ultimately you should listen to your health care provider for supplementation guidance.

Risks associated with a vitamin D deficiency during pregnancy include baby's increased risk for developing asthma and type 2 diabetes, and a higher incidence of cavities when baby is older. Deficiency is also associated with an increased risk of preterm labor and for developing preeclampsia. It is an easy nutrient to replenish if you are deficient, so it is wise to know your status. In the absence of deficiency, it is not advised to supplement with high amounts of this fat-soluble vitamin, so do not start mega-dosing on vitamin D pills on your own.

Month 5: Hitting the Halfway Point

At this stage, you may feel your baby moving around, doing its baby gymnastics this month. Few things are as exciting as feeling your baby kick for the first time. Your baby is starting to hear, so read a book or have a little conversation with your little one. Your baby will start to recognize your voice even before it's born. How cool is that?

Mom should focus on antioxidant intake this month to support health and combat the increased oxidative stress that may naturally occur during pregnancy. Foods that contain natural antioxidants include butternut squash, walnuts, avocado, berries, and black beans.

Calcium continues to be an important nutrient to protect your bone health and support baby's growing skeleton. Cheese is loaded with bone-building calcium, as well as muscle-building protein. Make sure you are choosing pasteurized varieties, especially for softer cheeses like Brie or feta. If you avoid dairy, make sure you choose nondairy alternatives like almond milk that is fortified with calcium to fill the gap. Other calcium-rich foods include almonds and green leafy vegetables. Try to avoid eating iron-rich foods (like beef) at the same time as you are enjoying calcium-rich foods, as both may compete for absorption.

Also, like last month, magnesium is an important nutrient to focus on, especially if you are experiencing leg cramps. Avocados, almonds, and beans are great sources of magnesium.

Foods like chicken will help support baby's nutrition needs. Between the high-quality protein, choline, and vitamin B_{12} naturally found in this food, it is a versatile and perfect choice during the fifth month of pregnancy.

Micronutrients like folate continue to be important for baby's development, and dark lettuces like romaine are great sources. Make sure that any lettuce you consume is washed very well and there are no recalls active.

Heartburn may strike this month. Some pregnant people swear that milk helps these symptoms subside, while others simply avoid acidic and spicy food to find relief. If you happen to take a calcium-rich antacid for relief, do not take them at the same time as you take an iron supplement. It is suggested to space these out at least two hours apart for best results.

WHAT TO EXPECT THIS MONTH

How Baby Is Developing: You may begin to feel your baby moving inside your belly. Your baby's muscles are forming, and hair may start to grow on your baby's head.

Changes in Mom: You may experience trouble sleeping, increased hunger, growing breasts, heartburn, runny nose/congestion, and leg cramps. Some mothers will also develop a linea nigra (a dark vertical line that goes down a pregnant mama's belly).

Foods to Enjoy: Cheese, butternut squash, walnuts, avocado, berries, chicken, black beans, and greens like lettuce.

Month 5 Sample Meal Plan

This month requires a focus on fruits, veggies, nuts, seeds, beans, and other antioxidant-rich foods. This meal plan is loaded with a balance of sweet and savory snacks to satisfy any craving you may have.

	BREAKFAST	LUNCH	DINNER	SNACK/ DESSERT
DAY 1	Popeye's Protein Breakfast Bowl (page 73)	Tomato stuffed with skipjack tuna salad with sliced cucumbers and 1 plum	Butternut Squash Mac and Cheese (page 76) with green salad	Vanilla frozen yogurt topped with almonds and cherries
DAY 2	Whipped Cottage Cheese Berry Bowl (page 68)	Leftover Butternut Squash Mac and Cheese (page 76) with sliced fresh cucumbers	Cobb Salad (page 74) with dried apricots	Peanut Butter Fruit Dip with Apples (page 92)
DAY 3	Leftover Popeye's Protein Breakfast Bowl	Leftover Cobb Salad and 1 apple	Creamy Bacon-and-Mushroom Chicken Bake (page 81) over ½ cup brown rice	Seasoned Snack Mix (page 90)
DAY 4	Leftover Whipped Cottage Cheese Berry Bowl	Leftover Creamy Bacon-and-Mushroom Chicken and rice	Fish Taco Baja Bowls (page 82)	Leftover Peanut Butter Fruit Dip with Apples
DAY 5	Avocado and Sweet Potato Toast (page 72)	Leftover Fish Taco Baja Bowls and 1 nectarine	Kitchen Sink Kale Salad (page 75)	Apple with cashew butter
DAY 6	Sweet Potato Pancakes (page 69) and Chicken-Apple Breakfast Sausages (page 71)	Leftover Kitchen Sink Kale Salad	Mediterranean-Inspired Stuffed Sweet Potatoes (page 78)	Leftover Seasoned Snack Mix
DAY 7	Leftover Sweet Potato Pancakes and leftover Chicken-Apple Breakfast Sausages	Triple Green Pesto Pasta (page 77)	Leftover Mediterranean-Inspired Stuffed Sweet Potatoes	Maple-Quinoa Bark (page 94)

Gestational diabetes is a condition that affects 6 to 9 percent of pregnant people. To receive a diagnosis of this condition, a test is conducted between weeks 24 and 28 of pregnancy.

During pregnancy, certain hormones are elevated in the body. Some hormones may cause insulin resistance, a condition in which glucose (sugar) is not absorbed into the cells as efficiently as it was before pregnancy. If you happen to be diagnosed with gestational diabetes, you should not assume that there has been any harm to your baby. With gestational diabetes, limiting concentrated sweets (think sugary sodas, candy, cookies), eating a fiber-rich diet, and monitoring portion sizes can all help manage blood sugar. Moderate exercise may help manage gestational diabetes as well.

Many people find that combining foods that contain carbohydrates, fiber, and healthy fats or protein are tolerated well when managing gestational diabetes. So, if you wish to enjoy a carbohydrate-rich apple, combining it with a tablespoon of nut butter may result in better blood glucose tolerance when compared with just eating the apple on its own.

If you do receive this diagnosis, following your doctor's and dietitian's advice is important to protect your baby from outcomes such as the baby being born too large or to protect yourself from things like high blood pressure. Gestational diabetes goes away once baby is born and often can be managed through dietary changes with the assistance of a registered dietitian or certified diabetes educator.

Month 6: Hello, Bump!

You may start to feel more than gentle kicks as you embark on your sixth month of pregnancy. At this point, there is likely no hiding the fact that you are pregnant, and your baby bump is popping out. Make sure to take some pictures.

Your iron needs may increase at this stage of pregnancy to support the increased volume that your blood needs to reach to support a growing blood supply. Eating iron-rich foods like spinach and beef can help support these needs. Your doctor may recommend an iron supplement. While taking this pill can help, it can cause constipation. You may have to try different remedies to find what works best for your own body, but here are two that have worked for some people: taking your iron supplement with food and eating probiotic-rich foods like yogurt or sauerkraut.

When focusing on iron-rich foods, combining them with vitamin C–rich foods such as oranges and grapefruit will enhance absorption. This interaction is important to focus on when consuming non-heme sources of iron like green leafy vegetables and beans. Iron that comes from a heme source like beef is often well-absorbed and doesn't need the additional vitamin C help.

If you are continuing to consume a small amount of caffeine, this may affect iron absorption. Do not eat iron-rich foods or take your iron supplement with your morning cup of joe if you want to maximize absorption.

If you are suffering from bloating, eating foods that are rich in potassium such as avocados, bananas, kiwis, and pistachios may help. Also, staying hydrated may help keep bloating at bay. Just keep in mind that you may be mistaking your baby bump as true bloat!

Baby's brain continues to be a focus and eating DHA-rich foods like salmon and shrimp helps fuel the little body with this important omega-3 fatty acid. If you aren't a seafood eater, it is important to take a DHA supplement to bridge the nutrient gap. Other nutrients that are going to support baby's brain this month include choline (egg yolks and peanuts) and healthy fats (avocado and walnuts).

Yogurt is a calcium-rich food that also provides protein and probiotics, or live bacteria that may offer a benefit to the host. Some data suggests that pregnant people who consume certain probiotics during pregnancy reduce the risk of their baby developing eczema after birth.

WHAT TO EXPECT THIS MONTH

How Baby Is Developing: Baby's eyelids begin to part, allowing eyes to open. Baby's lungs are now developed, but not quite ready to function on their own. Sucking reflexes continue to develop, and vital organs continue to become prepared for survival outside the womb.

Changes in Mom: Mom may experience fuzzy memory (aka "pregnancy brain"), bloating, increased appetite, swollen ankles, stretch marks on belly and thighs, darker nipples, and increased urination frequency.

Foods to Enjoy: Avocado, chocolate, salmon, watermelon, spinach, almonds, yogurt, and citrus.

Month 6 Sample Meal Plan

This month's meal plan focuses on a powerhouse combo of nutrients: folate, magnesium, healthy fats, protein, and more! You will find a variety of flavors in this meal plan, and each choice serves a purpose in terms of your healthy pregnancy journey. Note: This meal plan may help manage gestational diabetes in some cases and could be used as a guide until you meet with a health care provider.

	BREAKFAST	LUNCH	DINNER	SNACK/ DESSERT
DAY 1	Avocado and Sweet Potato Toast (page 72)	Fruit salad and ½ cup cottage cheese and almonds	Salmon, Broccoli, and Sweet Potato Sheet Pan (page 85)	Chocolate-Avocado Mousse (page 95)
DAY 2	Egg Muffin Cup (page 70) with 1 cup chopped watermelon	Leftover Salmon, Broccoli, and Sweet Potato Sheet Pan	Triple Green Pesto Pasta (page 77)	Leftover Chocolate-Avocado Mousse
DAY 3	Whipped Cottage Cheese Berry Bowl (page 68) (sub almonds for walnuts)	Leftover Triple Green Pesto Pasta	Blended Mushroom Burger with Oven-Baked Green Bean Fries (page 79)	Whole grain pita points with hummus and carrot sticks
DAY 4	Leftover Egg Muffin Cup with 1 small orange	Leftover Blended Mushroom Burger with Oven-Baked Green Bean Fries	Creamy Coconut-Lentil Dal (page 80) over ½ cup whole grain	Maple-Quinoa Bark (page 94)
DAY 5	Leftover Whipped Cottage Cheese Berry Bowl (sub almonds for walnuts)	Leftover Creamy Coconut-Lentil Dal with ½ cup whole grain and 1 orange	Herbed Lamb with Cauliflower Mash (page 88)	Seasoned Snack Mix (page 90)
DAY 6	Super Spiced Choco-Latte (page 67) and 1 leftover Egg Muffin Cup	Leftover Herbed Lamb with Cauliflower Mash	Chili-Lime Cod (page 84) with steamed veggies	Leftover Maple-Quinoa Bark
DAY 7	Sweet Potato Pancakes (page 69) with 1 teaspoon maple syrup and ½ cup berries	Leftover Chili-Lime Cod with whole wheat wrap, lettuce, and tomato with 1 small orange	Butternut Squash Mac and Cheese (page 76)	Leftover Seasoned Snack Mix

Super Spiced Choco-Latte

DAIRY-FREE, GLUTEN-FREE

SERVES 2

PREP TIME: 5 minutes / **COOK TIME:** 5 minutes

Enjoy every ounce of this hot chocolate packed with anti-inflammatory superfoods like collagen, ginger, and coconut oil. Oat milk has a natural sweetness and is rapidly growing in popularity. Because oats are a galactagogue (a food that supports breast milk production), this is a great recipe to continue making during your postpartum season. Substitute the same amount of another milk as you wish.

2 cups plain unsweetened oat milk

1 tablespoon coconut oil

1 tablespoon collagen peptides

2 tablespoons cacao powder

1 teaspoon ground ginger

1 teaspoon ground cinnamon

1 teaspoon pure vanilla extract or vanilla bean powder

1 teaspoon coconut sugar (optional)

Dash salt

1. In a small saucepan over medium heat, warm the oat milk and coconut oil. Add the collagen and stir to dissolve.

2. Add the cacao powder and stir until dissolved.

3. Carefully pour the warm mixture into a blender. Add the ginger, cinnamon, vanilla, coconut sugar (if using), and salt and blend for 15 seconds until frothy. Pour into a mug and serve immediately.

Ingredient tip: Collagen peptides are short-chain amino acids naturally derived from collagen protein (ideally from pasture-raised, grass-fed cattle), and they are a simple, healing protein powder with a neutral taste.

Per serving: Calories: 248; Total Fat: 11g; Saturated Fat: 7g; Cholesterol: 0mg; Sodium: 237mg; Carbohydrates: 31g; Fiber: 6g; Protein: 11g

Whipped Cottage Cheese Berry Bowl

GLUTEN-FREE, VEGETARIAN

SERVES 2

PREP TIME: 5 minutes

Whenever I hear complaints from clients about cottage cheese, it's solely because of the texture. But when it's whipped, cottage cheese takes on a completely different profile. If you can find cultured, probiotic-rich cottage cheese, this easy morning dish becomes a living recipe, rich in friendly gut bacteria, calcium, protein, and blood-sugar balancing cinnamon.

1 cup cultured whole-milk
   cottage cheese

½ cup blackberries

½ teaspoon ground cinnamon

¼ cup walnut pieces

¼ cup unsweetened shredded coconut

1. In a food processor or blender, blend the cottage cheese, blackberries, and cinnamon for 1 to 2 minutes, or until smooth and whipped.

2. Spoon the whipped cottage cheese mixture into two bowls and top with walnuts and coconut. Serve immediately.

3. Store in an airtight container in the refrigerator for up to 2 days.

Prep tip: If you prefer, whip only the cottage cheese and sprinkle the berries on top instead. You can also experiment with other low-glycemic fruit, such as raspberries or strawberries.

Per serving: Calories: 314; Total Fat: 23g; Saturated Fat: 11g; Cholesterol: 30mg; Sodium: 456mg; Carbohydrates: 14g; Fiber: 5g; Protein: 18g

Sweet Potato Pancakes

NUT-FREE, VEGETARIAN, FREEZER-FRIENDLY

SERVES 4

PREP TIME: 10 minutes / **COOK TIME:** 20 minutes

These pancakes come with a boost of beta-carotene from the sweet potatoes, which help support baby's developing eyes. Using real eggs gives these pancakes a choline and high-quality protein boost that both mom and baby benefit from. Enjoy these pancakes topped with fruit, pure maple syrup, or your favorite toppings.

1¼ cups reduced-fat milk

1¼ cup whole wheat flour

½ cup mashed cooked sweet potato

2 large eggs

2 teaspoons baking powder

1 teaspoon ground cinnamon

½ teaspoon vanilla extract

¼ teaspoon salt

6 teaspoons butter

1. In a large bowl, whisk together the milk, flour, sweet potato, eggs, baking powder, cinnamon, vanilla, and salt.

2. Heat a griddle or skillet over medium heat and add 2 teaspoons of butter.

3. Once melted, ladle ¾ cup of the batter onto the hot griddle. When the pancake begins to bubble after 2 to 3 minutes, flip with a spatula and continue cooking until golden brown, about 3 minutes.

4. Transfer to a plate. Repeat with the remaining butter and batter, until all the batter is used up.

Ingredient tip: For an extra boost of protein, add collagen peptides into your batter or top with nut butter. Once cool, freeze leftover pancakes for a quick-and-easy breakfast for busy days. If you don't have a cooked sweet potato handy, canned pumpkin can be used as a sub for another beta-carotene-rich option that is equally delicious.

Per serving: Calories: 287; Total Fat: 11g; Saturated Fat: 6g; Cholesterol: 115mg; Sodium: 516mg; Carbohydrates: 39g; Fiber: 5g; Protein: 11g

Egg Muffin Cups

GLUTEN-FREE, NUT-FREE, VEGETARIAN, FREEZER-FRIENDLY

MAKES 12 MUFFIN CUPS

PREP TIME: 10 minutes / **COOK TIME:** 20 minutes

This quick breakfast option is loaded with a slew of nutrients that help you start your day on the right foot. From the choline in the egg yolks to the calcium in the cheese, think of these egg muffin cups as mini multivitamins to complement your healthy lifestyle. Cook these up over a weekend and keep them in an airtight container in the refrigerator for a convenient breakfast option.

Nonstick cooking spray

6 large eggs

¼ cup shredded cheddar cheese

Salt

1 cup chopped fresh kale, stemmed

1 red bell pepper, diced

1. Preheat the oven to 350°F and spray a standard muffin tin with nonstick cooking spray.

2. In a medium bowl, beat the eggs. Mix in the cheese, season with salt, and set aside.

3. Divide the kale and bell pepper evenly among the muffin cups.

4. Pour in the beaten egg and cheese mixture, leaving ¼ inch at the top.

5. Bake for 20 minutes, or until cooked and golden on top.

Storage tip: Muffins can be stored in an airtight container in the refrigerator for 5 days or in the freezer for up to 2 months. Vegetable options can be swapped based on whatever you have on hand—mushrooms, spinach, or olives are all good choices.

Per serving (1 muffin cup): Calories: 51; Total Fat: 4g; Saturated Fat: 1g; Cholesterol: 96mg; Sodium: 48mg; Carbohydrates: 1g; Fiber: <1g; Protein: 4g

Chicken-Apple Breakfast Sausages

GLUTEN-FREE, NUT-FREE, FREEZER-FRIENDLY

MAKES 8 SAUSAGES

PREP TIME: 5 minutes / **COOK TIME:** 10 minutes

If you're looking to start your day with more protein and heme iron, these homemade breakfast sausages fit the bill. Try ground dark meat turkey instead of ground chicken for another yummy option.

1 pound ground chicken

3 tablespoons unsweetened applesauce

¾ teaspoon salt

½ teaspoon freshly ground black pepper

½ teaspoon garlic powder

½ teaspoon dried oregano

½ teaspoon dried basil

2 tablespoons ghee or grass-fed butter

1. In a large bowl, mix together the chicken, applesauce, salt, pepper, garlic powder, oregano, and basil until thoroughly incorporated.

2. Using your hands, form 8 patties that are about ½-inch thick.

3. In a skillet, heat the ghee over medium heat. Add the patties and cook for 3 to 4 minutes on each side, until cooked through.

4. Serve immediately.

Storage tip: Refrigerate in an airtight container for up to 3 days or freeze for up to 2 weeks. Place small squares of parchment paper between each sausage before freezing to prevent them from sticking together.

Per serving (1 patty): Calories: 114; Total Fat: 8g; Saturated Fat: 4g; Cholesterol: 60mg; Sodium: 228mg; Carbohydrates: 1g; Fiber: 0g; Protein: 10g

Avocado and Sweet Potato Toast

DAIRY-FREE, GLUTEN-FREE, VEGETARIAN

SERVES 2

PREP TIME: 5 minutes / **COOK TIME:** 5 minutes

You'll hear me sing praises to eggs throughout this book. Eggs are the most concentrated food source of choline, and this nutrient protects against neural tube defects. The sweet potatoes are bursting with beta-carotene, which is extra necessary for proper development of baby's face and features, and is a good source of magnesium, which is important for baby's bone development during this trimester.

1 sweet potato, cut into ¼-inch slices

1 teaspoon coconut oil

2 large eggs

1 avocado, pitted, peeled, and sliced

Sea salt

Freshly ground black pepper

1. Set a toaster to high and toast the sweet potato slices as you would slices of bread. Additional toasting will be required. You should be able to easily pierce the flesh with a fork.

2. In a small skillet, melt the coconut oil over medium heat. Crack the eggs into the skillet and scramble lightly as the eggs cook.

3. Divide the sweet potato between two plates. Layer the avocado over the toasts. Arrange the eggs on top and season with salt and pepper to taste.

Cooking tip: If the sweet potatoes are sliced too thin, they may burn quickly. Because every toaster is different, start out with ¼-inch slices and check their firmness with a fork after each round of toasting until cooked through. Do not insert a fork directly into the toaster.

Per serving: Calories: 318; Total Fat: 20g; Saturated Fat: 6g; Cholesterol: 187mg; Sodium: 89mg; Carbohydrates: 26g; Fiber: 8g; Protein: 10g

Popeye's Protein Breakfast Bowl

GLUTEN-FREE, NUT-FREE, VEGETARIAN

SERVES 6

PREP TIME: 10 minutes / **COOK TIME:** 10 minutes

Make way for plant-based iron! By now you know that heme iron found in animal foods is the fastest and most absorbable way to increase iron stores, but non-heme iron is effective, too, especially when you get it from spinach, arugula, or another leafy green.

1 cup canned black beans, rinsed and drained

1 cup water

2 teaspoons butter

1 zucchini, diced

½ cup fresh or frozen corn

2 cups chopped fresh spinach or arugula

4 large eggs

½ cup grated Parmesan cheese

1 avocado, pitted, peeled, and sliced

2 scallions, both white and green parts, sliced

Dash salt

Freshly ground black pepper

1. In a small saucepan, bring the beans and water to a boil over high heat. Reduce the heat to a simmer and cook for 5 minutes. Set aside.

2. In a small skillet over low heat, melt the butter. Add the zucchini and corn and cook for about 5 minutes, until lightly browned. Add the spinach and allow to wilt.

3. In a small bowl, whisk the eggs and pour them in the skillet. Scramble until cooked soft, about 2 minutes. Stir in the Parmesan.

4. Drain the beans and divide among six bowls. Top with the egg-and-vegetable mixture, avocado, and scallions. Season with salt and pepper.

Cooking tip: If you prefer your greens raw, toss the spinach or arugula with a little lemon juice and olive oil before adding to the breakfast bowls. When choosing your black beans, select ones that come in a can that is free from BPA lining.

Per serving: Calories: 163; Total Fat: 9g; Saturated Fat: 2g; Cholesterol: 112mg; Sodium: 140mg; Carbohydrates: 14g; Fiber: 6g; Protein: 10g

Cobb Salad

GLUTEN-FREE

SERVES 4

PREP TIME: 25 minutes

A classic Cobb salad can be full of ingredients that are not-so-great choices for a pregnant person. I swapped out some ingredients to make this popular salad nourishing and satisfying. It checks all the boxes: healthy fats, lean protein, and important vitamins and minerals. Simply pair it with a piece of fruit or a whole grain roll, and you will have a balanced meal in minutes!

⅔ cup extra-virgin olive oil

⅓ cup red wine vinegar

1 tablespoon Dijon mustard

¼ teaspoon salt

Freshly ground black pepper

1 head romaine lettuce, chopped

4 hard-boiled eggs, peeled and chopped

1 cup cooked diced chicken breast

8 nitrate- and nitrite-free bacon slices, cooked and crumbled

1 avocado, pitted, peeled, and thinly sliced

¾ cup cherry tomatoes, halved

1 cup shredded cheddar cheese

¾ cup chopped walnuts (optional)

1. In medium bowl, whisk the olive oil, vinegar, mustard, salt, and pepper.

2. On large platter or individual plates, place the romaine lettuce. Add the eggs, chicken, bacon, avocado, cherry tomatoes, and cheese in rows.

3. Drizzle with the dressing, and sprinkle with walnuts (if using).

Substitution tip: Swap out the chicken for cooked shrimp to get extra DHA. Bottled salad dressing can be used in place of homemade. Just make sure the one you choose isn't loaded with sugar or sodium. Feel free to sub turkey bacon instead of the traditional pork version.

Per serving: Calories: 714; Total Fat: 62g; Saturated Fat: 14g; Cholesterol: 230mg; Sodium: 874mg; Carbohydrates: 13g; Fiber: 6g; Protein: 29g

Kitchen Sink Kale Salad

GLUTEN-FREE, NUT-FREE, VEGETARIAN

SERVES 4

PREP TIME: 15 minutes

Dinosaur kale, also known as Lacinato or Tuscan kale, is more tender than curly and red kale, making it a perfect choice for this raw salad; however, the salad will be delicious whichever type you use. Kale offers more calcium than a cup of milk, so eat a lot to help fill up your reserves before birth and breastfeeding commence.

2 fresh kale bunches, stemmed and leaves ripped into bite-size pieces

1 avocado, pitted, peeled, and sliced, divided

1 roasted sweet potato, cubed

½ cup blueberries

3 scallions, both white and green parts, sliced

3 tablespoons hemp seeds

4 tablespoons plain whole-milk yogurt

2 tablespoons sunflower butter

1 tablespoon fresh lemon juice

1 teaspoon curry powder

1 teaspoon ground cumin

½ teaspoon salt

¼ teaspoon garlic powder

Freshly ground black pepper

1 teaspoon water, plus more as needed (optional)

1. In a large bowl, using your hands, massage the kale and half of the avocado until the kale begins to soften and the avocado is creamy, about 5 minutes.

2. Add the sweet potato, blueberries, scallions, and hemp seeds and toss together.

3. In a small bowl, make the dressing by stirring together the yogurt, sunflower butter, lemon juice, curry powder, cumin, salt, garlic powder, and pepper until well combined. Add water 1 teaspoon at a time if the dressing is too thick.

4. Toss the dressing with the salad and serve immediately. Top with the remaining avocado slices.

Ingredient tip: To make this recipe dairy-free, swap the dairy yogurt for a plant-based one. Make sure it isn't sweetened or flavored and choose the least processed one possible.

Per serving: Calories: 309; Total Fat: 16g; Saturated Fat: 2g; Cholesterol: 2mg; Sodium: 318mg; Carbohydrates: 34g; Fiber: 7g; Protein: 12g

Butternut Squash Mac and Cheese

NUT-FREE, VEGETARIAN, FREEZER-FRIENDLY

SERVES 4

PREP TIME: 15 minutes / **COOK TIME:** 30 minutes

Including butternut squash in this classic comfort food brings it up a notch in the nutrition department. Whole grain pasta provides some fiber to help add bulk to a pregnant mama's diet.

½ medium butternut squash, peeled, seeded, and chopped

1 tablespoon extra-virgin olive oil

8 ounces whole grain elbow macaroni

2 cups reduced-fat milk, divided

1 tablespoon butter

2 tablespoons all-purpose flour

⅛ teaspoon ground nutmeg

1 cup shredded aged white cheddar cheese

1 cup shredded sharp cheddar cheese

½ teaspoon salt

½ teaspoon freshly ground black pepper

1. Preheat the oven to 400°F.

2. On a baking sheet, spread the butternut squash in a single layer. Drizzle with olive oil and bake for 25 minutes, turning halfway through.

3. Bring a large pot of water to a boil and cook the macaroni according to the package directions. Rinse under cold water and set aside.

4. In a food processor, blend the butternut squash and ½ cup of milk and puree until smooth.

5. In large skillet, melt the butter over medium heat. When the butter is melted, whisk in the flour. Add the nutmeg and continue whisking. Add the remaining 1½ cups of milk and whisk until the mixture is smooth. Heat for about 10 minutes, until the sauce has thickened.

6. Turn the heat to low and stir in the butternut squash mixture.

7. Stir in the pasta and cheeses until melted and combined, about 2 minutes.

8. Season with salt and pepper

Per serving: Calories: 590; Total Fat: 29g; Saturated Fat: 15g; Cholesterol: 73mg; Sodium: 751mg; Carbohydrates: 61g; Fiber: 8g; Protein: 26g

Triple Green Pesto Pasta

GLUTEN-FREE, VEGETARIAN

SERVES 4

PREP TIME: 10 minutes / **COOK TIME:** 10 minutes

Getting those greens in when pregnant can feel daunting, but not when you make this flavorful pesto. It's bursting with purifying green herbs that gently support mama's liver. Add some spinach if you want to amp up the folate, vitamins K and A, and magnesium. You won't even notice it's there.

8 ounces chickpea pasta

½ cup chopped fresh parsley

½ cup chopped fresh cilantro

½ cup chopped fresh basil

½ cup extra-virgin olive oil

⅓ cup shelled unsalted sunflower seeds

¼ cup grated Parmesan cheese

2 tablespoons coconut butter

2 teaspoons fresh lemon juice

2 teaspoons white wine vinegar

½ teaspoon garlic powder

¼ teaspoon salt

Freshly ground black pepper

1. Bring a large pot of water to a boil and cook the pasta according to the package directions. Drain and keep warm in the pot.

2. Meanwhile, in a food processor, blend the parsley, cilantro, basil, and olive oil for 15 seconds, scraping down the sides with a silicone spatula.

3. Add the sunflower seeds, Parmesan, coconut butter, lemon juice, vinegar, garlic powder, salt, and pepper. Pulse until everything is incorporated. It won't be smooth.

4. Add the pesto to the pasta and toss until entirely covered. Serve immediately.

5. The pesto can be stored in an airtight container in the refrigerator for up to 6 days or in the freezer for up to 4 months.

Ingredient tip: I used chickpea pasta here to keep the carbs low while keeping the protein and fiber high. Use the pasta of your choice if that's not an issue for you. Feel free to sub the coconut butter with butter.

Per serving: Calories: 552; Total Fat: 41g; Saturated Fat: 13g; Cholesterol: 5mg; Sodium: 383mg; Carbohydrates: 47g; Fiber: 12g; Protein: 19g

Mediterranean-Inspired Stuffed Sweet Potatoes

DAIRY-FREE, GLUTEN-FREE, VEGETARIAN
SERVES 4
PREP TIME: 5 minutes / **COOK TIME:** 35 minutes

Sweet potatoes nourish the body and heal inflammation with their many nutrients, such as beta-carotene (the inactive form of vitamin A), and vitamins B_6 and C. Their higher fiber and complex carbohydrate count make sweet potatoes a great carb choice when you're tempted to grab less-nutritious options like breads or cereals.

4 medium sweet potatoes

2 tablespoons avocado oil

½ onion, diced

2 garlic cloves, minced

1 (15-ounce) can chickpeas, rinsed
   and drained

½ red bell pepper, diced

½ teaspoon dried oregano

¼ teaspoon dried parsley

¼ teaspoon salt

1 large avocado, pitted, peeled,
   and sliced

¼ cup pumpkin seeds

Juice of 1 lemon

1. Preheat the oven to 400°F.

2. Using a fork, poke each sweet potato 5 to 6 times. Place them on a baking sheet and bake for 30 minutes, or until cooked through.

3. Meanwhile, warm the avocado oil in a skillet over medium heat.

4. Add the onion and garlic and cook for 5 minutes until softened. Add the chickpeas, bell pepper, oregano, parsley, and salt. Stir well and cook for about 7 minutes, until heated through. Remove from the heat.

5. Remove the potatoes from the oven and cut each one lengthwise, almost through to the bottom. Squeeze each potato to create an opening for the filling.

6. Spoon equal amounts of the filling inside each potato. Top each with sliced avocado, pumpkin seeds, and a drizzle of lemon juice and serve.

Per serving: Calories: 397; Total Fat: 16g; Saturated Fat: 2g; Cholesterol: 0mg; Sodium: 232mg; Carbohydrates: 56g; Fiber: 14g; Protein: 11g

FREEZER-FRIENDLY, NUT-FREE

SERVES 4

PREP TIME: 10 minutes / **COOK TIME:** 15 minutes

Iron needs increase as pregnancy progresses, and beef is an excellent source of this important nutrient. However, beef does tend to be high in saturated fat. Making a blended burger with mushrooms balances this out.

Nonstick cooking spray

2 cups fresh green beans, trimmed

1 tablespoon all-purpose flour

¾ cup bread crumbs

2 tablespoons grated Parmesan cheese

2 tablespoons extra-virgin olive
  oil, divided

8 ounces washed button
  mushrooms, diced

8 ounces ground beef

2 large eggs, divided

3 tablespoons ground flaxseed

Salt

Freshly ground black pepper

4 whole grain buns

4 iceberg lettuce leaves

1 tomato, sliced

4 teaspoons yellow mustard (optional)

1. Preheat the oven to 425°F. Spray a baking sheet with cooking spray.

2. Toss the green beans in the flour. In a medium bowl, combine the bread crumbs, cheese, and ½ teaspoon of salt. In a shallow baking dish, beat the remaining egg. Dip the green beans in the egg, then into the breadcrumb mixture. Place the coated green beans in a layer on the sheet and bake for 12 minutes or until golden brown.

3. Meanwhile, in a medium pan, heat 1 tablespoon of olive oil over medium heat. Sauté the mushrooms for about 4 minutes until golden brown. Remove from the pan and cool for a few minutes.

4. In a medium bowl, combine the mushrooms, beef, 1 egg, flaxseed, and salt and pepper to taste and form into 4 patties. In the same pan, heat the remaining tablespoon of olive oil over medium heat. Cook the burgers for 10 minutes, flip, and then cook until the desired doneness is achieved (I recommend at least 165°F). Serve on buns topped with lettuce, tomato, and mustard (if using) and a side of green beans.

Per serving: Calories: 559; Total Fat: 25g; Saturated Fat: 6g; Cholesterol: 146mg; Sodium: 540mg; Carbohydrates: 54g; Fiber: 9g; Protein: 32g

Creamy Coconut-Lentil Dal

DAIRY-FREE, GLUTEN-FREE

SERVES 4

PREP TIME: 5 minutes / **COOK TIME:** 20 minutes

Worried about hypertension and high blood pressure? Work on increasing your potassium intake by eating dishes like this one that include high-potassium plant sources, such as lentils, spinach, and squash. If using store-bought broth, be aware of the potentially higher sodium content and consider not adding any more salt.

1 tablespoon coconut oil

3 cups diced butternut squash

½ onion, diced

3 cups Slow Cooker Beef Bone Broth (page 87) or store-bought

1 cup red lentils, rinsed and drained

1 cup minced fresh spinach

1 (5-ounce) can coconut cream

2 teaspoons brown mustard

2 teaspoons fresh lemon juice

½ teaspoon salt

½ teaspoon ground turmeric

½ teaspoon ground cumin

1. In a large pot, melt the coconut oil over medium heat. Add the squash and onion and cook for 5 minutes, until the onion is translucent.

2. Add the broth, lentils, spinach, coconut cream, mustard, lemon juice, salt, turmeric, and cumin and bring to a boil. Cover, reduce the heat to a simmer, and cook for 10 minutes, until the lentils are tender.

3. Ladle into bowls and serve warm.

Serving tip: This dal can be eaten as a main course or as a side with chicken, fish, or vegetables. Try topping it with Greek yogurt, fresh herbs, or toasted pine nuts.

Per serving: Calories: 523; Total Fat: 29g; Saturated Fat: 25g; Cholesterol: 0mg; Sodium: 600mg; Carbohydrates: 50g; Fiber: 12g; Protein: 20g

Creamy Bacon-and-Mushroom Chicken Bake

GLUTEN-FREE, NUT-FREE

SERVES 6

PREP TIME: 10 minutes / **COOK TIME:** 6 to 8 hours

This recipe tastes best made with real heavy cream, which—because it has less lactose and more fat than whole milk—may be more digestible for those who are sensitive to dairy.

½ teaspoon dried oregano

1 teaspoon salt, divided

½ teaspoon freshly ground black
  pepper, divided

¼ teaspoon dried thyme

¼ teaspoon dried basil

¼ teaspoon dried rosemary

¼ teaspoon dried sage

4 bone-in, skin-on chicken thighs

2 tablespoons butter, divided

2½ cups sliced white mushrooms

1 cup heavy cream

6 nitrate- and nitrite-free bacon slices,
  cooked and chopped

1 teaspoon garlic powder

1. Preheat the oven to 350°F.

2. In a small bowl, combine the oregano, ½ teaspoon of salt, ¼ teaspoon of pepper, the thyme, basil, rosemary, and sage. Sprinkle onto both sides of the chicken.

3. In a cast-iron skillet, melt 1 tablespoon of butter over medium-high heat. Add the chicken thighs and cook for 1 to 2 minutes per side. Transfer the skillet to the oven and bake for 20 minutes, until the chicken is cooked through and the juices run clear. Remove from the oven, transfer the chicken to a plate, and set aside.

4. Carefully return the skillet to the stovetop. Melt the remaining 1 tablespoon of butter over medium-high heat. Add the mushrooms and cook until soft, about 5 minutes.

5. Add the cream, bacon, garlic powder, remaining ½ teaspoon of salt, and remaining ¼ teaspoon of pepper. Stir and bring to a simmer. Return the chicken to the skillet, stir, and cook until warmed through.

6. Spoon onto plates and serve hot.

Per serving: Calories: 440; Total Fat: 39g; Saturated Fat: 19g; Cholesterol: 151mg; Sodium: 715mg; Carbohydrates: 3g; Fiber: 1g; Protein: 20g

Fish Taco Baja Bowls

DAIRY-FREE, GLUTEN-FREE, NUT-FREE

SERVES 4

PREP TIME: 10 minutes / **COOK TIME:** 20 minutes

Tilapia is a low-mercury fish that's easy to come by in most markets. Like most fish, it brings a good amount of vitamin D, vitamin B$_{12}$, and protein to the table. Using premade cauliflower rice keeps the carbohydrate content of this dish down.

½ teaspoon chili powder

½ teaspoon salt

½ teaspoon garlic powder

¼ teaspoon ground cumin

4 (4-ounce) tilapia fillets

1 teaspoon avocado oil

1 red bell pepper, thinly sliced

½ red onion, thinly sliced

1 cup corn

4 cups shredded green cabbage

2 cups cooked cauliflower rice

1 cup cooked black beans, rinsed
  and drained

1 avocado, pitted, peeled, and quartered

2 tablespoons fresh lime juice

1. In a small bowl, combine the chili powder, salt, garlic powder, and cumin. Sprinkle evenly over both sides of the fish.

2. In a cast-iron skillet, heat the avocado oil over medium heat. Add the fish and cook for 3 to 4 minutes per side, until cooked through. Transfer the fish to a plate and set aside.

3. Using the same skillet over medium-high heat, cook the bell pepper, onion, and corn for about 5 minutes, stirring often, until the onion is translucent.

4. Add the cabbage, cauliflower rice, and beans to the skillet, mix to combine, then divide among four bowls. Place a fish fillet over the vegetables in each bowl. Top each with a quarter of the avocado and sprinkle with the lime juice.

Cooking tip: Most grocery stores now sell frozen cauliflower rice. Be sure to thaw and lightly cook the cauliflower in a skillet before adding to this dish.

Per serving: Calories: 333; Total Fat: 11g; Saturated Fat: 2g; Cholesterol: 56mg; Sodium: 335mg; Carbohydrates: 34g; Fiber: 12g; Protein: 31g

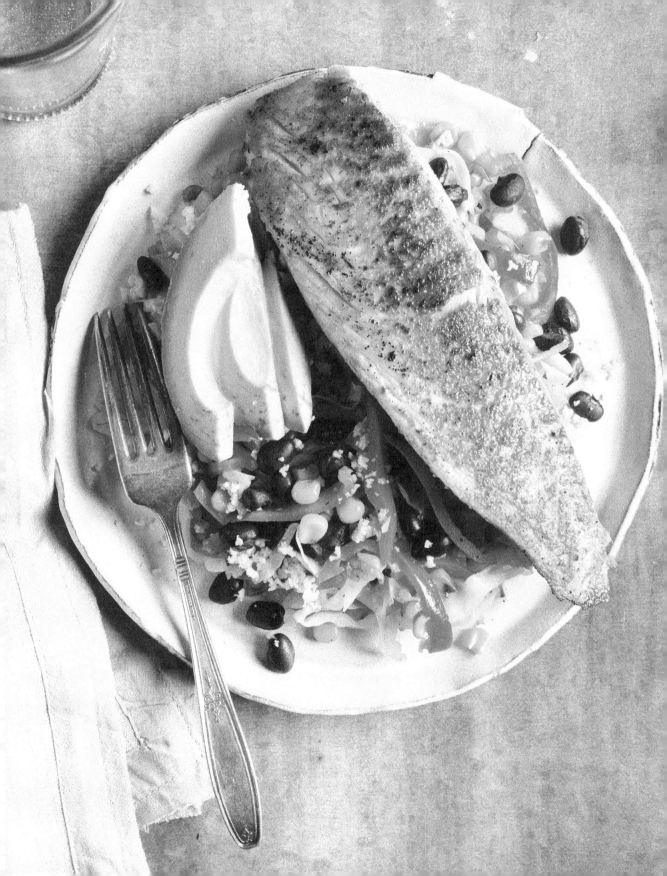

Chili-Lime Cod

GLUTEN-FREE, NUT-FREE

SERVES 4

PREP TIME: 30 minutes / **COOK TIME:** 12 minutes, plus 20 minutes to chill

Seafood is the richest source of iodine, which is one of the many reasons I encourage healthy fish consumption during pregnancy. Cod is considered low in mercury and is therefore safe to consume during pregnancy. The high omega-3 fatty acids in cod also bring you closer to your DHA and EPA intake goals.

1 teaspoon dried oregano

1 teaspoon chili powder

1 teaspoon garlic powder

½ teaspoon salt

½ teaspoon ground cumin

Freshly ground black pepper

4 cod fillets (about 14 ounces total)

1 tablespoon extra-virgin olive oil

2 tablespoons ghee, melted

4 tablespoons fresh lime juice

1. In a small bowl, combine the oregano, chili powder, garlic powder, salt, cumin, and pepper.

2. Line a baking sheet with parchment paper and place the fillets on the baking sheet. Brush them with the olive oil and sprinkle the spice mixture over the top.

3. Refrigerate the baking sheet with the cod for at least 20 minutes or up to 8 hours.

4. Preheat the oven to 450°F.

5. Bake the fillets for 12 minutes, until the fish reaches an internal temperature of 130°F.

6. Place a fillet on each of four plates, drizzle with the ghee and lime juice, and serve.

Serving tip: For a balanced meal, serve over cauliflower rice with your favorite roasted non-starchy vegetable.

Per serving: Calories: 185; Total Fat: 12g; Saturated Fat: 5g; Cholesterol: 54mg; Sodium: 348mg; Carbohydrates: 3g; Fiber: 1g; Protein: 18g

Salmon, Broccoli, and Sweet Potato Sheet Pan

DAIRY-FREE, GLUTEN-FREE, NUT-FREE

SERVES 4

PREP TIME: 10 minutes / **COOK TIME:** 30 minutes

Salmon is one of the best foods for pregnancy. The natural fatty acids found in this fish help support baby's eye and brain development and may ward off development of post-partum depression. The sweet potatoes are loaded with tons of nutrients that help support both mom and baby. Make sure to keep the skin on to give yourself an extra boost of fiber to keep constipation at bay.

Nonstick cooking spray

2 sweet potatoes, cut into wedges

¼ cup extra-virgin olive oil, plus more for drizzling

1 teaspoon minced garlic

½ teaspoon salt

Freshly ground black pepper

4 cups chopped broccoli florets

4 (4-ounce) skinless salmon fillets

1 tablespoon honey

1. Preheat the oven to 400°F. Spray a baking sheet with cooking spray and place in the oven.

2. In a bowl or plastic bag, mix the sweet potatoes with the olive oil, garlic, salt, and pepper.

3. Place the potatoes on the baking sheet and cook for 15 minutes.

4. Take the sheet pan out of the oven, add the broccoli, and place the salmon on top. Drizzle the salmon with olive oil and sprinkle with pepper. Drizzle the honey on top of the salmon. Bake for 15 minutes, or until the salmon is cooked through.

Substitution tip: If you don't care for broccoli, Brussels sprouts or cauliflower can be used instead. Halibut can be used in place of salmon.

Per serving: Calories: 348; Total Fat: 18g; Saturated Fat: 3g; Cholesterol: 55mg; Sodium: 521mg; Carbohydrates: 22g; Fiber: 4g; Protein: 25g

Nutrient-Dense Bolognese

GLUTEN-FREE, NUT-FREE, FREEZER-FRIENDLY

SERVES 6

PREP TIME: 10 minutes / **COOK TIME:** 30 minutes

This is my favorite way to incorporate nutrient-dense liver into my diet without losing out on taste. Although a classic Bolognese is traditionally cooked for hours to allow the flavors to meld together, this delectable and healthy version can be ready to eat in half an hour!

2 tablespoons ghee or grass-fed butter

½ cup chopped yellow onion

3 garlic cloves, minced

⅔ cup chopped celery

⅔ cup chopped carrot

1 pound ground beef (preferably grass-fed)

3 ounces beef liver, trimmed of any connective tissue and finely chopped

1 (14-ounce) can diced tomatoes

1 tablespoon white wine vinegar

⅛ teaspoon ground nutmeg

Dash salt

Dash freshly ground black pepper

Cooked pasta of choice, for serving

1. In a large skillet, heat the ghee over medium heat. Add the onion and garlic and cook for 5 minutes, stirring occasionally. Add the celery and carrot and cook for another 5 minutes, stirring occasionally.

2. Push the vegetables to the side of the skillet. Add the ground beef and liver and cook for about 10 minutes, using a spoon to break up the meat as it cooks.

3. Add the tomatoes and their juices, vinegar, nutmeg, salt, and pepper and bring to a simmer.

4. Serve over pasta or spaghetti squash.

5. Store the sauce in an airtight container in the refrigerator up to 4 days or in the freezer for up to 4 months.

Per serving: Calories: 385; Total Fat: 13g; Saturated Fat: 6g; Cholesterol: 97mg; Sodium: 127mg; Carbohydrates: 46g; Fiber: 7g; Protein: 26g

Slow Cooker Beef Bone Broth

DAIRY-FREE, GLUTEN-FREE, NUT-FREE

MAKES ABOUT 4 QUARTS

PREP TIME: 5 minutes / **COOK TIME:** 8 to 24 hours

I wish I could give jars of this broth to every pregnant person I know. This recipe makes use of bones that are often tossed out, even though they are immensely rich in healing and powerful nutrients like collagen, glycine, protein, iron, and zinc.

2 pounds beef marrow bones

2 carrots, roughly chopped

½ onion, roughly chopped

1 celery stalk, roughly chopped

3 garlic cloves, roughly chopped

2 bay leaves

1 tablespoon apple cider vinegar

1. In a slow cooker, combine the beef marrow bones, carrot, onion, celery, garlic, bay leaves, and vinegar. Add enough filtered water to cover all the ingredients.

2. Set the slow cooker to high and cook for at least 8 hours and up to 24 hours. The longer it simmers, the more nutrients will effectively leach into the broth.

3. Skim off and discard any foam that may have formed on the surface. Strain the broth through a fine-mesh sieve or cheesecloth and store in glass containers with lids.

4. The broth can be stored in the refrigerator for up to 1 week or in the freezer for up to 5 months. Bring it to a boil before consuming.

Cooking tip: Roasting the bones beforehand will greatly enhance the flavor of the finished broth. Place the bones in a roasting pan and roast at 400°F for 40 to 60 minutes. Drain off any fat and start at the beginning of the recipe.

Per serving (1 cup): Calories: 30; Total Fat: 0g; Saturated Fat: 0g; Cholesterol: 0mg; Sodium: 97mg; Carbohydrates: 2g; Fiber: 0g; Protein: 5g

Herbed Lamb with Cauliflower Mash

GLUTEN-FREE, NUT-FREE

SERVES 4

PREP TIME: 10 minutes / **COOK TIME:** 10 minutes

Try to choose grass-fed lamb, which has been shown to have a far better ratio of omega-3s to omega-6s than conventionally raised lamb. Because your baby's brain is 60 percent fat, specifically DHA, the more omegas, the merrier. Purple and other colored cauliflower have a higher antioxidant content than white cauliflower. If it's in season where you live, give it a try!

4 (4-ounce) lamb chops

1 teaspoon salt, divided

½ teaspoon freshly ground black pepper

2 tablespoons avocado oil

1 teaspoon dried rosemary

4 thyme sprigs, minced

1 large cauliflower head, broken into small florets

1 tablespoon ghee or grass-fed butter

½ teaspoon garlic powder

1. Season the lamb all over with ¾ teaspoon of salt and the pepper.

2. In a large skillet, heat the avocado oil, rosemary, and thyme over medium-high heat. Add the lamb chops to the pan, making sure they are not touching.

3. Sear for 5 minutes, spooning avocado oil from the bottom of the pan over the chops halfway through. Flip the chops and sear for another 5 minutes. Remove from the heat and allow to rest for 5 minutes.

4. Meanwhile, place the cauliflower in a pot. Fill with enough water to cover the florets by 1 inch, bring to a boil, and cook for 10 minutes until tender.

5. Drain the pot, then place the cauliflower in a food processor along with the ghee, garlic powder, and the remaining ¼ teaspoon of salt. Pulse to combine, then blend until smooth.

6. To serve, spoon the cauliflower mash onto plates and arrange the lamb next to it. Serve warm.

Ingredient tip: If you don't like cauliflower, you can make the mash with celery root or rutabaga.

Per serving: Calories: 410; Total Fat: 31g; Saturated Fat: 12g; Cholesterol: 89mg; Sodium: 620mg; Carbohydrates: 12g; Fiber: 6g; Protein: 24g

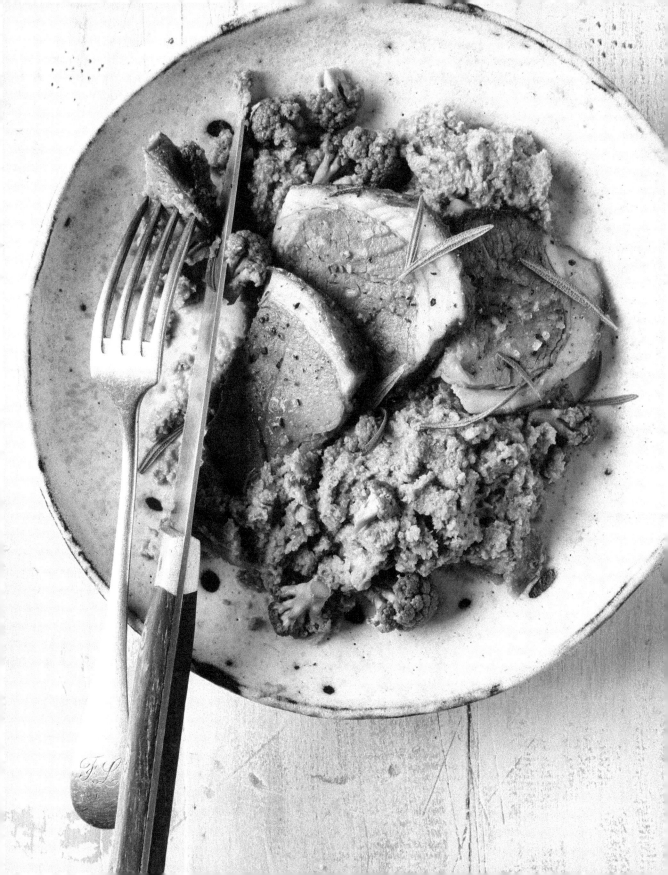

Seasoned Snack Mix

DAIRY-FREE, GLUTEN-FREE, VEGETARIAN

SERVES 12

PREP TIME: 5 minutes / **COOK TIME:** 20 minutes

Most nuts and seeds are fantastic sources of folate, magnesium, zinc, and non-heme iron, not to mention protein. If you're feeling hungry or a little hypoglycemic, keep some of this seasoned savory snack mix close by.

1 cup unsalted sliced almonds

1 cup unsalted cashews

1 cup unsalted pecans

1 cup unsalted pumpkin seeds

1 cup unsalted shelled sunflower seeds

2 tablespoons coconut oil, melted

⅓ cup nutritional yeast

1 teaspoon chili powder

½ teaspoon paprika

½ teaspoon salt

¼ teaspoon garlic powder

¼ teaspoon onion powder

1. Preheat the oven to 325°F. Line a baking sheet with parchment paper.

2. In a large bowl, combine the almonds, cashews, pecans, pumpkin seeds, and sunflower seeds and toss with the coconut oil.

3. Spread the nuts in single layer on the baking sheet.

4. In a small bowl, combine the nutritional yeast, chili powder, paprika, salt, garlic powder, and onion powder. Sprinkle over the nut mixture evenly.

5. Bake for 15 to 20 minutes, until lightly browned and crispy.

6. Store in an airtight container at room temperature for 5 to 7 days.

Ingredient tip: Sprouted nuts, if you can find them, are a great way to add extra nutrients that are more bioavailable and more easily absorbed by your body.

Per serving: Calories: 320; Total Fat: 27g; Saturated Fat: 5g; Cholesterol: 6mg; Sodium: 87mg; Carbohydrates: 13g; Fiber: 5g; Protein: 12g

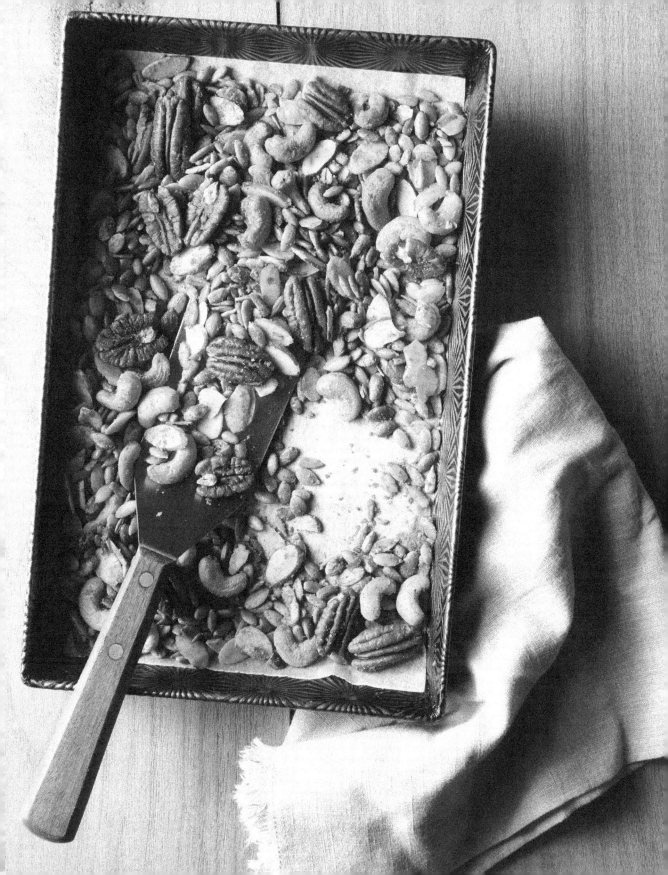

Peanut Butter Fruit Dip with Sliced Apples

GLUTEN-FREE, VEGETARIAN

SERVES 4

PREP TIME: 10 minutes

We all know that fruit is a great snack during pregnancy but eating a plain apple or pear day in and day out can get pretty monotonous. Eating fruit with a homemade dip can bring excitement to an otherwise ho-hum snack. Combining peanut butter and yogurt adds some fat and protein to the fruit to make the snack more satiating than eating the fruit on its own. Feel free to use the dip as an oatmeal topping in the morning, too!

½ cup natural smooth peanut butter

¼ cup plain whole-milk yogurt or coconut milk–based yogurt

1 teaspoon pure maple syrup

2 medium apples, cut into wedges

1. In small bowl, stir together the peanut butter, yogurt, and maple syrup.

2. Serve the sliced apples with the dip.

Substitution tip: Top the dip with mini dark chocolate chips for some extra sweetness, or some dried coconut flakes for a tropical twist. Swap the apple for any firm fruit. Strawberries or sliced pears work well in this recipe.

Per serving: Calories: 249; Total Fat: 17g; Saturated Fat: 3g; Cholesterol: 2mg; Sodium: 10mg; Carbohydrates: 21g; Fiber: 5g; Protein: 9g

Ranch Zucchini Chips

DAIRY-FREE, GLUTEN-FREE, NUT-FREE, VEGETARIAN

SERVES 4

PREP TIME: 10 minutes / **COOK TIME:** 1 hour 30 minutes

Here is your new go-to pregnancy snack when you're craving the crunch of a zesty potato chip (or those irresistible Cool Ranch Doritos!). I love zucchini for their B vitamin, fiber, and mineral content. Go ahead and make this recipe even if you don't have all the spices listed. A little garlic powder and salt can be quite satisfying.

2 zucchini, thinly cut into coins

2 teaspoons garlic powder

2 teaspoons onion powder

1 teaspoon dried oregano

1 teaspoon dried parsley

1 teaspoon dried dill

½ teaspoon dried chives

½ teaspoon salt

Freshly ground black pepper

1 tablespoon avocado oil

1. Preheat the oven to 225°F. Line a baking pan with parchment paper.

2. Pat the zucchini coins with paper towels to draw out excess moisture.

3. In a small bowl, mix the garlic powder, onion powder, oregano, parsley, dill, chives, salt, and pepper.

4. In a large bowl, toss the zucchini with the avocado oil. Sprinkle in the seasonings, making sure to coat each piece as evenly as possible.

5. Place in a single layer on the baking sheet. Bake for 90 minutes, until completely dried out and crispy, checking at the 1-hour mark. Let cool to room temperature before serving.

Cooking tip: Use a mandoline, if you have one, to get the zucchini coins extra thin. The thinner the slices, the faster they'll cook.

Per serving: Calories: 57; Total Fat: 4g; Saturated Fat: 0g; Cholesterol: 0mg; Sodium: 246mg; Carbohydrates: 6g; Fiber: 1.5g; Protein: 1.5g

Maple-Quinoa Bark

DAIRY-FREE, VEGETARIAN, FREEZER-FRIENDLY

SERVES 12

PREP TIME: 10 minutes / **COOK TIME:** 25 minutes

This recipe is an easy take on traditional brittle that will help satisfy your pregnant sweet tooth. I've intentionally included several sweet treats and snacks in this book because so many people crave sugar at some point in their pregnancy. Start by choosing a source of sweetness that also includes some vitamins and minerals in its unrefined state (like the maple syrup used here) and be sure to include a balance of proteins and fats, as this recipe highlights.

½ cup cooked quinoa

½ cup chopped unsalted peanuts

¼ cup rolled oats

2 tablespoons ground flaxseed

2 tablespoons chia seeds

2 tablespoons coconut oil

½ cup pure maple syrup

Dash salt

1. Preheat the oven to 325°F. Grease a baking pan or sheet pan.

2. In a medium bowl, mix together the quinoa, peanuts, oats, flaxseed, and chia seeds. Set aside.

3. In a small saucepan over medium heat, melt the coconut oil, add the maple syrup, and mix together.

4. Fold into the quinoa and peanut mixture.

5. Spread the mixture onto the pan in a thin layer. Bake for 25 minutes, checking halfway to make sure the edges aren't burning. If it is, fold the outer edges of the mixture into the center of the pan and continue to cook. Let cool completely before cutting into 12 pieces. Season with salt.

Storage tip: Wrap the bark in parchment paper, place in an airtight container, and store in the freezer for up to 3 months.

Per serving (1 piece): Calories: 121; Total Fat: 7g; Saturated Fat: 3g; Cholesterol: 0mg; Sodium: 23mg; Carbohydrates: 14g; Fiber: 2g; Protein: 3g

Chocolate-Avocado Mousse

DAIRY-FREE, GLUTEN-FREE, VEGETARIAN

SERVES 4

PREP TIME: 10 minutes, plus 2 hours chill time

Sometimes we need some decadence in our diet, and chocolate mousse fits the bill. Using ripe avocados in the recipe gives this dessert a healthy dose of monounsaturated fats, fiber, antioxidants, and loads of vitamins and minerals like folate to support a healthy pregnancy. Enjoy this as a dessert or a midday treat if a chocolate craving strikes. Nobody ever said you have to avoid treats when you are expecting—even if you are managing gestational diabetes!

2 very ripe avocados, pitted and peeled

½ cup bittersweet chocolate, melted

¼ cup unsweetened cocoa powder

¼ cup plain unsweetened almond milk

2 tablespoons pure maple syrup

2 teaspoons vanilla extract

Berries, for garnish (optional)

1. In food processor, blend the avocados, chocolate, cocoa powder, almond milk, maple syrup, and vanilla until creamy.

2. Divide among four bowls and chill covered for at least 2 hours.

3. Garnish with berries (if desired).

Cooking tip: For an extra indulgent addition, top with a dollop of fresh whipped cream and a sprinkle of chocolate chips. During the summertime, try freezing the mousse into ice pop molds for a frozen chocolate treat!

Per serving: Calories: 315; Total Fat: 21g; Saturated Fat: 9g; Cholesterol: 0mg; Sodium: 19mg; Carbohydrates: 32g; Fiber: 9g; Protein: 5g

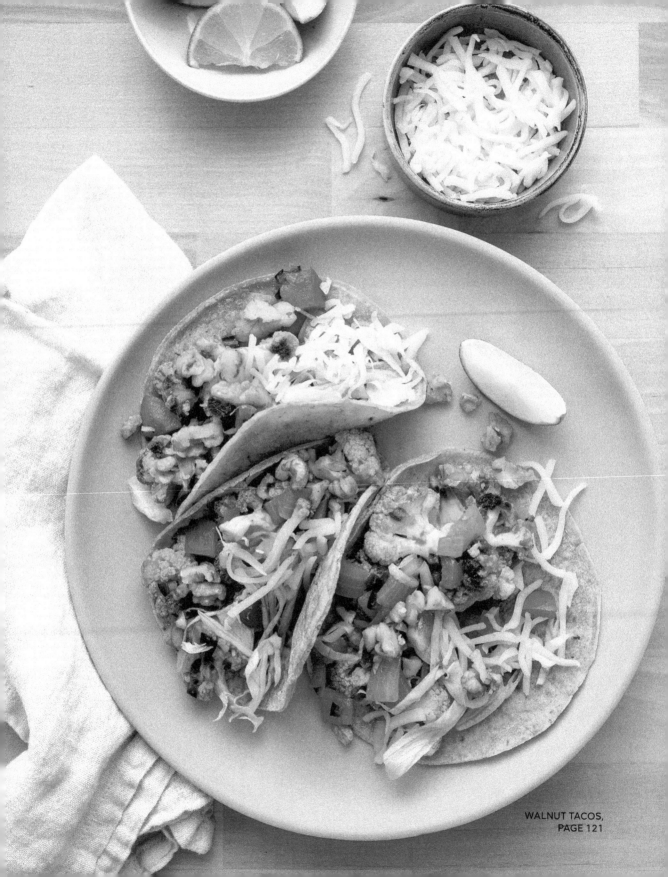

WALNUT TACOS,
PAGE 121

The Third Trimester

You are in the home stretch of your pregnancy and you can look forward to holding your little bundle of joy very soon. Your belly is likely getting bigger, your appetite is getting stronger, and you are making the final preparations before your new little addition arrives. Welcome to your third trimester, mama. You are almost there!

During the third trimester, don't let nutrition fall to the wayside. Make sure that you are eating a variety of foods that contain different nutrients to help ensure that you and your baby are getting everything you both need. Some general tips include: Keep taking your prenatal vitamin, eat your fruits and veggies, eat low-mercury seafood twice a week, and stay hydrated. A little effort on the nutrition front can go a long way.

Month 7: Entering the Third Trimester

Your baby is storing more fat to get it ready for life outside the womb. Unfortunately, if you have been coasting in terms of symptoms during your second trimester, know that some symptoms may return or appear during the last few months of pregnancy.

Make sure you are taking in enough iron to help support your growing body. Iron-rich foods like beef, kale, and even raisins can help you meet your iron needs. Health care providers can check iron status relatively easy during a prenatal visit to confirm whether additional iron is needed. Eat a healthy dose of vitamin C–rich foods like oranges with your iron foods to help support ample absorption.

Protein needs are higher than before you became pregnant, and high-quality protein like chicken should be on the menu.

Foods like peanuts are a pregnancy superfood, especially during this month. The manganese naturally found in these legumes aids in the growth of fetal tissue and bone. It is also helpful in preventing premature contraction of the uterus, and the natural vitamin E helps mom support a healthy blood pressure.

Baby's brain is continuing to grow and eating foods like shellfish can help supply the body with brain-boosting nutrients like DHA, iodine, and selenium. Eating seafood twice a week will help you meet the need for these important nutrients. Not a seafood fan? Brazil nuts, nori snacks, and eggs can help, too.

You may want to avoid fizzy drinks like seltzers and sodas during the third trimester. Drinking bubbles may result in indigestion.

Niacin is key for the healthy growth of your baby. Brown rice, mushrooms, and chicken will all provide you with niacin and, in turn, help keep your baby's growth and development on track.

During the third trimester, your calorie needs may increase. A general recommendation is to aim for around 2,400 calories per day, but this number varies based on pre-pregnancy weight, how much weight has been gained thus far during pregnancy, and other factors. Many experts recommend eating around 450 calories more than before pregnancy. Again, the focus is on nutrient-dense foods that provide vitamins and minerals, healthy fats, protein, and carbohydrates.

General dietary recommendations do not vary significantly from those given during the second trimester. Here is what is recommended as a daily intake:

2 or 3 servings of lean protein, or at least 75 grams of protein

3 or more servings of whole grains

4 or 5 servings of fruits and vegetables (more veggies than fruit preferably)

4 servings of calcium-rich food like dairy, almonds, and tofu

At least 1 serving of a healthy fat, like nuts

WHAT TO EXPECT THIS MONTH

How Baby Is Developing: Your baby is developing more brain tissue, storing more fat, and working on breathing. Muscles and lungs continue to mature, and fingernails and toenails are developing as well.

Changes in Mom: Symptoms may include leg cramps, insomnia, frequent urination, heartburn, constipation and gas, swollen ankles, leaking breasts, Braxton-Hicks contractions (false labor pains), and dry, flaky skin.

Foods to Enjoy: Kale, black beans, chicken, almonds, shellfish, oranges, yogurt, and peanuts.

Month 7 Sample Meal Plan

This month's meal plan focuses on foods that support baby's growth and development. Also, as mom's belly is growing and there is less "free space" for food, it highlights foods that pack a punch in the nutrition department without taking up a lot of real estate in the tummy. You will notice a variety of fruits are offered on this meal plan. Because staying hydrated is so important during pregnancy, enjoying fruit as a hydrating food as well as nourishment helps meet fluid needs.

	BREAKFAST	LUNCH	DINNER	SNACK/DESSERT
DAY 1	Apple-Cinnamon Overnight Oats with Collagen Peptides (page 108)	Tuna melt sandwich: 3 ounces skipjack tuna and pasteurized cheese on seeded bread with ½ banana	Mediterranean-Inspired Sheet Pan Chicken (page 124)	Air-popped popcorn sprinkled with 1 tablespoon chocolate chips
DAY 2	Banana Custard with Chia (page 111)	Leftover Mediterranean-Inspired Sheet Pan Chicken and ½ cup berries	Roasted Cauliflower Salad (page 117) with ½ cup whole grain	Frozen Yogurt Bark (page 137)
DAY 3	Leftover Apple-Cinnamon Overnight Oats with Collagen Peptides	Leftover Roasted Cauliflower Salad with 1 orange	Tomato and Feta Baked Cod (page 126) with ½ cup raspberries	Crispy Chili Chickpeas (page 135)
DAY 4	Banana Custard with Chia (page 111)	Leftover Tomato and Feta Baked Cod with ½ cup raspberries	Ground Turkey and Butternut Squash Chili (page 125)	Leftover Crispy Chili Chickpeas
DAY 5	Date with a Smoothie (page 112)	Leftover Ground Turkey and Butternut Squash Chili	Chicken with Dates (page 122) over ½ cup quinoa	Leftover Frozen Yogurt Bark
DAY 6	Eggs over Sweet Potato and Kale Hash (page 116)	Leftover Chicken with Dates over ½ cup quinoa	Spaghetti with Sardines and Greens (page 128)	Leftover Frozen Yogurt Bark
DAY 7	Leftover Eggs over Sweet Potato and Kale Hash	Leftover Ground Turkey and Butternut Squash Chili	Leftover Spaghetti with Sardines and Greens	Cherry tomato, olive, provolone cheese, and fresh basil skewer

At this point, your baby can stick out its tongue and taste amniotic fluid. If you aren't experiencing any gastrointestinal challenges like heartburn, try to eat a variety of flavorful foods from now on. From garlic to salmon, eating flavorful foods instead of sticking with bland standbys may predispose your baby to being more open to eating the familiar flavor later on. Data suggests that moms who ate a wide range of flavors had babies who were more open to eating different flavors. While there is no surefire way to prevent your future kiddo from living off macaroni and cheese with a side of chicken nuggets, eating a variety of foods during pregnancy certainly won't hurt.

If you are normally a ho-hum chicken eater, try eating some crab for a change. Instead of sticking with mild vegetables like carrots, try some radishes or Brussels sprouts to expose baby to a more unique flavor.

If your pregnancy is preventing you from eating a variety of foods, don't sweat it. It is more important to focus on foods that you can tolerate that will support a healthy pregnancy than forcing yourself to eat foods simply for the exposure.

For a super flavorful recipe, try out the Chicken with Dates (page 122) recipe. Feel free to add more spices for an extra boost of flavor!

Month 8: Feeding a Fully Developed Baby

Your eighth month of pregnancy is associated with lots of appointments, planning, and unfortunately, random people attempting to touch your belly and give you unsolicited advice. People are very excited for you and you may start celebrating with special gatherings to acknowledge the end of your pregnancy. At this point, it's entirely possible that you could be welcoming your little one into the world any day.

Your belly is getting bigger, which means less space in your tummy for food. Eat nutrient-dense foods that pack a punch instead of filler food with little to no nutritional value, like potato chips.

Omega-3 fatty acids are important for baby's brain and eye development, and these important nutrients have also been shown to provide mom with some benefits. From perinatal depression risk reduction to reducing inflammation, eating foods like low-mercury fish and shrimp can support both mom and baby during this month.

Foods like nuts, meats, and plant-based oils (such as olive and avocado oils) provide calories as well as important nutrients like folate, iron, and zinc—no empty calories here!

You may have trouble getting quality sleep right now. Between having a baby dancing on your bladder, a belly that prevents you from sleeping on your tummy, and side effects like heartburn, pregnancy insomnia is common. Foods that naturally contain melatonin like tart cherries may help you catch some zzz's safely.

Pantothenic acid is a B vitamin that performs many roles in the body, including helping break down carbohydrates, proteins, and fats. You need enough of this nutrient to make sure the macronutrients you are taking in are actually used and are supporting you and your baby. Foods that contain pantothenic acid include beans, meats, broccoli, poultry, and milk.

WHAT TO EXPECT THIS MONTH

How Baby Is Developing: Baby's major organs are functioning on their own except for the lungs. Bones are hardening. Baby continues to accumulate fat and grow.

Changes in Mom: Braxton-Hicks contractions, varicose veins, shortness of breath, exhaustion, decreased appetite due to your baby taking up so much space in your belly, feeling warm/hot flashes, mood swings, anxiety, blurry vision, hemorrhoids, and insomnia.

Foods to Enjoy: Oats, eggs, walnuts, apples, carrots, prunes, beef, vitamin D and calcium-fortified orange juice, and tart cherries.

Month 8 Sample Meal Plan

This meal plan is chock-full of foods that support your growing baby and growing belly. Meal ideas are simple, so you don't have to spend your precious energy in the kitchen. If you feel hungry while following this plan, honor your hunger and eat larger quantities or add a nutrient-dense snack (like whole grain crackers and nut butter). Now is not the time to fight hunger—if your body is telling you it needs more nutrition, listen. Enjoy your meals, kick your feet up, and relax into your final weeks of pregnancy.

	BREAKFAST	LUNCH	DINNER	SNACK/DESSERT
DAY 1	Blueberry Baked Oatmeal (page 109) with 1 cup orange juice	1 cup cooked chickpea pasta topped with broccoli, lemon juice, and pasteurized ricotta	Grilled Beef Kabobs with Brown Rice (page 132) with grilled pineapple	Homemade Granola Bar (page 133)
DAY 2	Avocado Deviled Eggs (page 115) with 1 small apple	Leftover Grilled Beef Kabobs with Brown Rice with ½ cup grapes	Warm Chicken Salad with Pears and Swiss Chard (page 118)	Nutty Energy Bites (page 134)
DAY 3	Leftover Blueberry Baked Oatmeal with 1 cup orange juice	Leftover Warm Chicken Salad with Pears and Swiss Chard	Minestrone (page 120) with green salad	Edamame tossed with lemon juice, chopped basil, rice vinegar, and olive oil
DAY 4	Leftover Avocado Deviled Eggs	Leftover Minestrone with 1 pear	Walnut Tacos (page 121) with black bean and corn salad	Leftover Homemade Granola Bars
DAY 5	Date with a Smoothie (page 112)	Leftover Walnut Tacos with 1 apple	Roasted Cauliflower Salad (page 117) with ½ cup berries	Nuts for Dates (page 136)
DAY 6	Almond Crust Quiche (page 110)	Leftover Roasted Cauliflower Salad with 1 nectarine	Slow Cooker Short Ribs (page 130) with celery root and parsnip mash	Guacamole with jicama sticks
DAY 7	Leftover Almond Crust Quiche	Leftover Slow Cooker Short Ribs with celery root and parsnip mash	Pan-Fried Lemon Butter Trout (page 127) with steamed veggies	Leftover Nuts for Dates

If you are planning on delivering in the hospital, it's a good idea to pack your hospital bag before you go into labor. While the hospital will likely offer you all the Jell-O you can eat, it may not offer you the best snacks to keep you fueled during your stay.

When you are in active labor, you will be limited with what you are allowed to eat. Keep that in mind when planning your snacks. Ask your health care provider if items like honey are okay to eat when you are in active labor, as every practitioner has their own protocols.

Some tips when packing snacks for your hospital bag include:

Dates and nut butter: if you can't get a full meal, snacking on dates filled with nut butter will help give your body a balance of fiber, protein, and healthy fats as well as satisfy a sweet tooth.

Dried fruit: Fiber will be key after baby is born, and fruit is a natural source. Keeping dried fruits on hand is a great way to meet your fiber needs without worrying about refrigeration.

Electrolyte drink: Staying hydrated post-labor is important, and natural energy drinks like coconut water or maple water can help keep fluids balanced. It's important that you only drink clear liquids during and after labor.

Gum: Your mouth may get super dry and you may be glad to have something to chew on while waiting for your baby's grand entrance. Chewing gum after a C-section may help get your bowels moving sooner, which means mama gets to eat sooner!

Honey sticks: You may not be allowed to eat any food until your baby is born once you are admitted. Labor requires a lot of energy, and honey is packed with carbohydrates for a quick burst of fuel. Because honey is considered a clear liquid, it is often okay to suck some down when food is off-limits, and it's well-tolerated, too!

Protein bars: Whether you plan on breastfeeding or bottle feeding or whether you gave birth via C-section or vaginally, you will need a lot of protein and calories for recovery and support. Having some protein bars stashed away can help you keep you fueled during a midnight feed or snuggle.

Month 9: Eating in the Final Stretch

Your skin continues to stretch as baby grows. Focusing on skin-supporting nutrients like protein and vitamin C can help support your changing skin. Don't forget to stay hydrated, too!

To support both yours and baby's bones, calcium intake continues to be important. Foods like almonds are a nutrient-dense source of calcium that are easy to snack on while resting or running to the doctor for a checkup.

Make sure you are still loading up on fiber and balancing it out with adequate fluids to prevent constipation. Constipation remains a concern post-baby for many people, so stay ahead of the game by fueling up with fruit, veggies, whole grains, and other fiber-rich foods now.

Fatigue can set in during your last month of pregnancy. Instead of loading up on caffeine, which is not recommended during pregnancy, focus on energy-supporting foods like whole grains and prunes. Whole grains contain manganese, which plays a part in helping fuel your body with organic energy. Prunes, on the other hand, are a sweet snack and have been shown to promote satiety. Unlike other foods with a higher glycemic index, prunes are digested and absorbed slowly by the body, which helps sustain energy over a longer period of time.

Biotin is a nutrient that you may think of to support healthy hair and nails, and it does the same for baby. Eating foods like cauliflower, carrots, and salmon will help provide your body with a boost of biotin.

WHAT TO EXPECT THIS MONTH

How Baby Is Developing: Your baby is growing and putting on fat to get ready for its life outside of the cozy and warm womb. Baby may be in a head-down position and ready to pass through the birth canal, or right-side up and in the breech position. Your birth plan should be discussed with your doctor, especially if baby is in the breech position.

Changes in Mom: Typical maternal health changes include Braxton-Hicks contractions, varicose veins, shortness of breath, exhaustion, constipation, heartburn, colored vaginal discharge (red or brown), and pelvic pain. Many of these symptoms are typical during this stage of pregnancy.

Foods to Enjoy: Sweet potato, watermelon, tofu, salmon, chia seeds, almonds, and kiwi.

Month 9 Sample Meal Plan

This final meal plan is loaded with food to support your last month of pregnancy. It focuses on easy foods to make sure both you and your baby are getting what is needed for the healthiest outcomes. You will notice it includes dates, a food that has been shown to support cervical ripening and may even help with labor! Enjoy your last month of pregnancy!

	BREAKFAST	LUNCH	DINNER	SNACK/ DESSERT
DAY 1	Salsa Verde Baked Eggs (page 114)	Grilled cheese sandwich with 1 kiwi	Spaghetti with Sardines and Greens (page 128)	Nuts for Dates (page 136)
DAY 2	Banana Custard with Chia (page 111)	Leftover Spaghetti with Sardines and Greens with ½ cup chopped melon	Minestrone (page 120)	Rice cakes topped with avocado and diced hard-boiled egg
DAY 3	Apple-Cinnamon Overnight Oats with Collagen Peptides (page 108)	Leftover Minestrone with 1 kiwi	Chicken with Dates (page 122) with ½ cup quinoa and green salad	Leftover Nuts for Dates
DAY 4	Date with a Smoothie (page 112)	Leftover Chicken with Dates with ½ cup quinoa, and a green salad	Warm Chicken Salad with Pears and Swiss Chard (page 118)	Homemade Granola Bars (page 133)
DAY 5	Leftover Apple-Cinnamon Overnight Oats with Collagen Peptides	Leftover Warm Chicken Salad with Pears and Swiss Chard with whole grain crackers	Pan-Fried Lemon Butter Trout (page 127) with ½ cup whole grains	Nutty Energy Bites (page 134)
DAY 6	Almond Crust Quiche (page 110) with 1 kiwi	Leftover Pan-Fried Lemon Butter Trout with 1 cup chopped watermelon	Grilled Beef Kabobs with Brown Rice (page 132)	Leftover Homemade Granola Bars
DAY 7	Leftover Almond Crust Quiche with 1 kiwi	Leftover Grilled Beef Kabobs with Brown Rice and ½ mango	Mediterranean-Inspired Sheet Pan Chicken (page 124)	Leftover Nutty Energy Bites

Apple-Cinnamon Overnight Oats with Collagen Peptides

NUT-FREE

SERVES 4

PREP TIME: 5 minutes, plus 2 hours to chill

....

Overnight oats are an easy make-ahead breakfast that you can grab on your way out the door in the morning. The addition of collagen peptides helps you meet your protein needs and gives your body a boost of important amino acids that may help support the growth of your baby's skin and collagen.

....

2 cups rolled oats

2 medium apples, shredded

2 cups reduced-fat milk

2 tablespoons pure maple syrup

2 tablespoons full-fat vanilla
  Greek yogurt

2 tablespoons chia seeds

2 tablespoons collagen peptides

2 teaspoons ground cinnamon

¼ teaspoon ground nutmeg

1. In a medium bowl, combine the oats, apples, milk, maple syrup, yogurt, chia seeds, collagen peptides, cinnamon, and nutmeg and mix well.

2. Place in mason jars and chill for at least 2 hours or overnight.

Substitution tip: If you are avoiding dairy, swap out the Greek yogurt and milk with vanilla coconut milk or vanilla almond milk—both will result in an equally delicious breakfast. Consider adding a scoop of protein powder, as many dairy alternatives don't contain comparable quantities of protein to dairy milk.

....

Per serving: Calories: 339; Total Fat: 7g; Saturated Fat: 2g; Cholesterol: 11mg; Sodium: 79mg; Carbohydrates: 57g; Fiber: 10g; Protein: 14g

Blueberry Baked Oatmeal

DAIRY-FREE, VEGETARIAN

SERVES 6

PREP TIME: 5 minutes / **COOK TIME:** 30 minutes

This baked oatmeal is a treat that will last for days in the refrigerator and is easy to change up with toppings like Greek yogurt, unsweetened jam, nut butters, or cottage cheese. By choosing rolled oats over quick oats, you're receiving more iron, protein, and fiber.

1 teaspoon coconut oil

2 cups rolled oats

¼ cup shredded unsweetened coconut

2 tablespoons coconut sugar

1½ teaspoons baking powder

1 teaspoon ground cinnamon

½ teaspoon ground ginger

½ teaspoon salt

1½ cups plain unsweetened almond milk

2 large eggs

½ teaspoon vanilla extract or vanilla bean powder

½ cup blueberries

1. Preheat the oven to 400°F. Grease an 8-by-10-inch baking dish with the coconut oil.

2. In a large bowl, stir together the oats, coconut, coconut sugar, baking powder, cinnamon, ginger, and salt and set aside.

3. In a separate bowl, whisk together the almond milk, eggs, and vanilla.

4. Add the egg mixture to the oat mixture and mix together. Add the blueberries and stir gently to combine.

5. Pour into the baking dish and bake for 30 minutes, until lightly browned and firm.

6. Let cool for 5 minutes and serve warm.

Ingredient tip: For a vegan alternative, combine 2 tablespoons of chia seeds with ⅓ cup of water and let sit for 15 minutes. Use this chia mixture to replace the eggs.

Per serving: Calories: 183; Total Fat: 7g; Saturated Fat: 2g; Cholesterol: 55mg; Sodium: 270mg; Carbohydrates: 26g; Fiber: 4g; Protein: 6g

Almond Crust Quiche

GLUTEN-FREE, VEGETARIAN

SERVES 6

PREP TIME: 10 minutes / **COOK TIME:** 31 minutes

. . . .

Almonds contain a significant amount of folate, magnesium, and calcium, as well as protein and fiber, making them the perfect base for this third-trimester breakfast treat. It also contains nutritional yeast, which is a deactivated yeast high in B vitamins that comes in powder form and has a nutty, cheesy, salty flavor.

. . . .

2 cups almond flour

9 large eggs, divided

2 tablespoons ghee, melted

1 teaspoon salt, divided

½ teaspoon garlic powder

2 cups chopped asparagus

1 medium zucchini, thinly sliced

½ cup shredded carrots

⅓ cup plain unsweetened almond milk

3 tablespoons nutritional yeast

Freshly ground black pepper

1. Preheat the oven to 375°F.

2. In a large bowl, mix together the almond flour, 1 egg, ghee, ½ teaspoon of salt, and the garlic powder until it comes together in a ball.

3. Press the dough into the bottom and sides of a standard pie plate, crimping the edges. Bake for 6 minutes. Remove the pie plate from the oven and set it on a wire rack. Leave the oven on.

4. Layer the asparagus, zucchini, and carrots in the crust. Set aside.

5. In a large bowl, whisk the remaining 8 eggs, almond milk, nutritional yeast, remaining ½ teaspoon of salt, and the pepper. Pour the mixture over the vegetables.

6. Bake for 25 minutes, until the eggs are firmly set.

7. Cut into wedges and serve.

Ingredient tip: Nutritional yeast is available at most grocery stores and is often found in bulk sections as well. It's sometimes referred to as "nooch" and is popular in the vegan community.

. . . .

Per serving: Calories: 254; Total Fat: 18g; Saturated Fat: 6g; Cholesterol: 290mg; Sodium: 148mg; Carbohydrates: 10g; Fiber: 6g; Protein: 18g

Banana Custard with Chia

DAIRY-FREE, GLUTEN-FREE, VEGETARIAN

SERVES 1

PREP TIME: 2 minutes, plus 20 minutes to chill

I love this easy breakfast for its smooth simplicity. Chia seeds contain an impressive amount of fiber for their small size, plus some plant-based omega-3 fatty acids, calcium, iron, magnesium, and potassium. Because they have such a great balance of soluble and insoluble fiber, they keep everything regular in the digestion department.

1 banana

⅓ cup full-fat coconut milk

2 tablespoons chia seeds

1. In a blender, blend the banana, coconut milk, and chia seeds for 1 minute.

2. Pour into an airtight container and refrigerate for 20 minutes before serving, or up to 12 hours, if you prefer to make it the night before.

Prep tip: If you'd like more texture, blend the banana and milk, transfer to your container, and stir in the chia seeds by hand before refrigerating.

Per serving: Calories: 427; Total Fat: 28g; Saturated Fat: 18g; Cholesterol: 0mg; Sodium: 18mg; Carbohydrates: 39g; Fiber: 15g; Protein: 8g

Date with a Smoothie

DAIRY-FREE, VEGETARIAN

SERVES 2

PREP TIME: 5 minutes

Studies have shown that when you consume dates in your last trimester, it can help you have an easier labor and birth. Just be sure to pair them with healthy fats and protein; this recipe contains generous portions of both, from the coconut milk, seeds, and nut butter.

1 cup full-fat coconut milk

1 banana

Handful ice

⅓ cup cooked oatmeal

3 Medjool dates, pitted

2 tablespoons hemp seeds

2 tablespoons chia seeds

1 tablespoon peanut butter

2 teaspoons unsweetened cocoa powder

½ teaspoon ground cinnamon

In a blender, blend the coconut milk, banana, ice, oatmeal, dates, hemp seeds, chia seeds, peanut butter, cacao powder, and cinnamon until smooth.

Ingredient tip: If you need to thin it out, add water a little at a time. You can also use a frozen banana instead of ice.

Per serving: Calories: 545; Total Fat: 38g; Saturated Fat: 25g; Cholesterol: 0mg; Sodium: 59mg; Carbohydrates: 45g; Fiber: 14g; Protein: 14g

Cinnamon-Apple Oat Muffins

VEGETARIAN

MAKES 12 MUFFINS

PREP TIME: 10 minutes / **COOK TIME:** 25 minutes

While the average person doesn't keep a pantry stocked with a variety of gluten-free flours, plain rolled oats are gluten-free and most people have them stored in a kitchen cabinet. In this recipe, you can quickly create oat flour using the same oats you use to make oatmeal.

1½ cups rolled oats

1 cup unsweetened applesauce

¼ cup almond butter

⅓ cup coconut sugar

1 cup full-fat coconut milk

1 egg

2 tablespoons grass-fed ghee

1 teaspoon pure vanilla extract or vanilla bean powder

1½ teaspoons ground cinnamon

1½ teaspoons baking powder

½ teaspoon baking soda

¼ teaspoon sea salt

1. Preheat the oven to 375°F. Line a 12-cup muffin tin with paper liners.

2. In a food processor, pulse the oats until a coarse flour forms. Transfer the oat flour to a small bowl and set aside.

3. In the food processor, blend the applesauce, almond butter, coconut sugar, coconut milk, egg, ghee, vanilla, cinnamon, baking powder, baking soda, and salt until smooth.

4. Slowly add the oat flour, pulsing until well combined.

5. Pour the batter into the lined muffin tins. Bake for 20 to 25 minutes, until a toothpick inserted into a muffin comes out clean.

6. Let cool for 5 minutes before serving.

7. Store in an airtight container at room temperature for up to 2 days or in the refrigerator for up to 1 week.

Cooking tip: To avoid waste, consider purchasing silicone muffin molds, which are nonstick, reusable, and washable.

Per serving (1 muffin): Calories: 172; Total Fat: 11g; Saturated Fat: 6g; Cholesterol: 19mg; Sodium: 101mg; Carbohydrates: 17g; Fiber: 2g; Protein: 3g

Salsa Verde Baked Eggs

DAIRY-FREE, GLUTEN-FREE, NUT-FREE, VEGETARIAN

SERVES 2

PREP TIME: 2 minutes / **COOK TIME:** 15 minutes

Getting your choline isn't get any easier than this! Grab your favorite green salsa (keep it mild if you've been experiencing heartburn). Choline still matters during the third trimester, especially for mom, as it supports liver function—and your liver is now wading through so many pregnancy hormones. A good amount of your choline intake is consumed by the baby, so keep including choline-rich foods in your diet to avoid maternal depletion.

1 cup salsa verde

4 large eggs

Sea salt

Freshly ground black pepper

1 avocado, sliced

1. Preheat the oven to 400°F.

2. In a small cast-iron skillet, pour in the salsa verde. Crack the eggs on top of the salsa. Season with salt and pepper.

3. Place the skillet into the oven and bake for 15 minutes until the eggs have set.

4. Transfer to plates and top with the avocado before serving.

Ingredient tip: If green salsa isn't your thing, try mild red salsa or even pesto.

Per serving: Calories: 300; Total Fat: 22g; Saturated Fat: 5g; Cholesterol: 327mg; Sodium: 836mg; Carbohydrates: 13g; Fiber: 6g; Protein: 14g

Avocado Deviled Eggs

GLUTEN-FREE, NUT-FREE, VEGETARIAN

SERVES 4

PREP TIME: 5 minutes, plus 1 hour chill time / **COOK TIME:** 10 minutes

Sour cream can be a great source of probiotics and healthy fats. But did you also know it's packed with calcium and the active form of vitamin A? This retinol is the form that's ready for your body to start using right away. Opt for cultured if you can find it to ensure the good bacteria are intact. Remember, when it comes to dairy products: the less processed, the better!

6 hard-boiled eggs, peeled

1 avocado, pitted and peeled

1 tablespoon Dijon mustard

1 tablespoon sour cream (preferably cultured)

½ tablespoon fresh lemon juice

½ teaspoon garlic powder

½ teaspoon salt

1. Cut each egg in half lengthwise. Remove the yolks and place them in a small bowl.

2. Scoop the avocado flesh into the bowl with the yolks.

3. Add the mustard, sour cream, lemon juice, garlic powder, and salt. Mash well with a fork and stir until the mixture becomes creamy.

4. Arrange the egg white halves on a plate. Spoon the yolk mixture into the egg whites. Refrigerate for 1 hour before serving.

Storage tip: Because of the avocado in this recipe, these don't store well. Plan to eat them the same day you make them.

Per serving: Calories: 177; Total Fat: 14g; Saturated Fat: 3g; Cholesterol: 247mg; Sodium: 376mg; Carbohydrates: 5g; Fiber: 3g; Protein: 9g

Eggs over Sweet Potato and Kale Hash

DAIRY-FREE, GLUTEN-FREE, NUT-FREE, VEGETARIAN

SERVES 4

PREP TIME: 5 minutes / **COOK TIME:** 30 minutes

Get a dose of vegetables first thing in the morning with this simple eggs-and-hash recipe. The fiber and nutrients will help mom feeling energized and satisfied all morning. Enjoying eggs during pregnancy supplies your little one with brain-supporting choline, iodine, and other important essential nutrients.

Nonstick cooking spray

1 cup chopped fresh kale

2 tablespoons extra-virgin olive
  oil, divided

4 large sweet potatoes

1 large white onion, diced

4 large eggs

1 tablespoon chopped fresh parsley

¼ teaspoon salt

1. Preheat the oven to 400°F. Spray the baking sheet with cooking spray.

2. Toss the kale with 1 tablespoon of olive oil.

3. On the prepared baking sheet, spread the sweet potato, onion, and kale in a single layer. Drizzle the remaining tablespoon of olive oil over the vegetables.

4. Bake for 20 minutes, stirring halfway.

5. Remove from the heat. Using a spoon, create four small spaces within the vegetables. Crack one egg into each hole. Bake for 10 minutes, or until the eggs are cooked through.

6. Remove from the oven and sprinkle with parsley and salt.

Cooking tip: If you like your eggs a bit runny, make sure to use pasteurized eggs to reduce the risk of foodborne illness. Any green leafy vegetable can be used in place of kale. Feel free to sprinkle pasteurized feta cheese on top of this dish for a flavor boost along with additional calcium and protein.

Per serving: Calories: 330; Total Fat: 12g; Saturated Fat: 3g; Cholesterol: 187mg; Sodium: 327mg; Carbohydrates: 45g; Fiber: 7g; Protein: 10g

Roasted Cauliflower Salad

DAIRY-FREE, GLUTEN-FREE, VEGETARIAN

SERVES 4

PREP TIME: 15 minutes / **COOK TIME:** 35 minutes

Cauliflower is a cruciferous vegetable bursting with excellent nutrients. It's loaded with vitamin C, an anti-inflammatory antioxidant that helps lower the risk of becoming group B strep–positive.

1 tablespoon coconut oil

1 cauliflower head, chopped

1 (15-ounce) can chickpeas, rinsed and drained

½ red onion, thinly sliced

1½ teaspoons ground cumin

1 teaspoon chili powder

¾ teaspoon salt

1 teaspoon garlic powder

¼ cup finely chopped fresh parsley

2 tablespoons fresh lemon juice

2 tablespoons extra-virgin olive oil

1. Preheat the oven to 450°F.

2. Place the coconut oil in a 9-by-13-inch baking pan and transfer to the oven to melt.

3. Remove from the oven and add the cauliflower, chickpeas, and onion and mix together.

4. In a small bowl, mix together the cumin, chili powder, salt, and garlic powder. Sprinkle the mixture over the vegetables in the baking pan and toss to coat.

5. Bake for 15 minutes, until the vegetables start to brown. Let cool slightly. Sprinkle with the parsley, add the lemon juice and olive oil, and toss to coat.

6. Serve warm.

Cooking tip: To save time, use precut frozen organic cauliflower (thawed before beginning recipe prep). To melt the coconut oil quickly, place it on the baking pan in the oven while it preheats.

Per serving: Calories: 350; Total Fat: 24g; Saturated Fat: 10g; Cholesterol: 35mg; Sodium: 390mg; Carbohydrates: 30g; Fiber: 9g; Protein: 9g

Warm Chicken Salad with Pears and Swiss Chard

DAIRY-FREE, GLUTEN-FREE

SERVES 6

PREP TIME: 10 minutes / **COOK TIME:** 10 minutes

Swiss chard is one of the most nutritious greens on the planet. Similar to beets, chard is high in betalains, which provide antioxidant, anti-inflammatory, and detoxification support, all crucial during pregnancy.

2 cups shredded cooked chicken

6 cups chopped Swiss chard

1 pear, sliced

4 mini peppers, sliced

¼ cup pine nuts, toasted

½ cup extra-virgin olive oil

1 shallot, minced

2 tablespoons fresh lemon juice

2 tablespoons apple cider vinegar

1 tablespoon Dijon mustard

¼ teaspoon salt

1. Preheat the oven to 350°F.

2. Wrap the shredded chicken in a piece of parchment paper, place it on the baking sheet, and warm for 10 minutes.

3. In a large bowl, combine the chard, pear, peppers, and pine nuts.

4. In a small bowl, whisk together the olive oil, shallot, lemon juice, vinegar, mustard, and salt.

5. Add the dressing to the salad and toss to combine.

6. Add the warm chicken to the bowl, toss well, and serve immediately.

Ingredient tip: Feel free to chop up the chard stems along with the leaves, though the stems are best cooked due to their high fiber and oxalic acid content.

Per serving: Calories: 295; Total Fat: 23g; Saturated Fat: 3g; Cholesterol: 36mg; Sodium: 217mg; Carbohydrates: 10g; Fiber: 3g; Protein: 16g

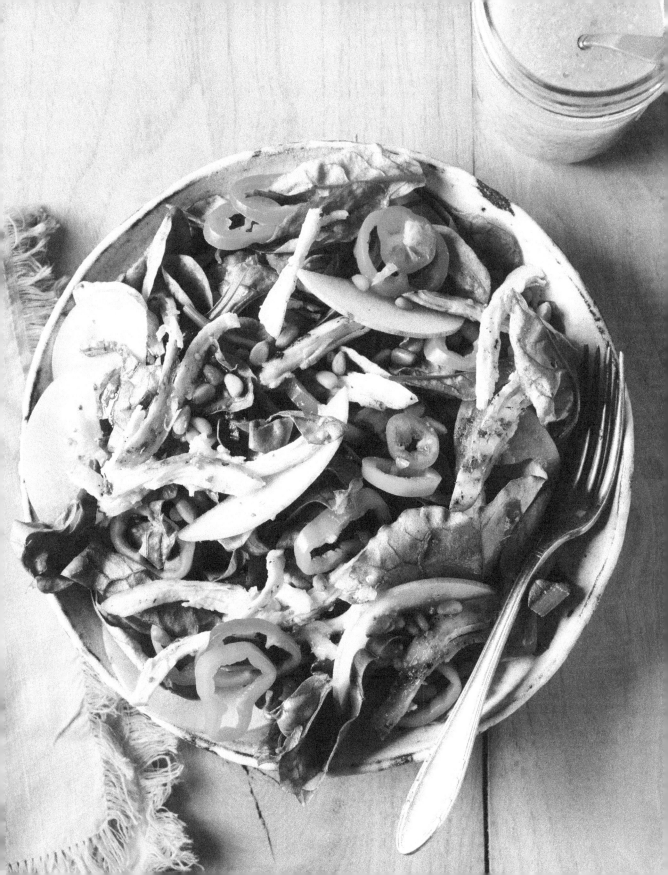

Minestrone

DAIRY-FREE, GLUTEN-FREE, NUT-FREE, VEGETARIAN, FREEZER-FRIENDLY

SERVES 4

PREP TIME: 10 minutes / **COOK TIME:** 15 minutes

As the final weeks draw near, it can get hard to fit food into your baby-filled tummy. Reach for easy-to-digest, simple recipes like this vegetable-based soup. It's a great way to sneak some nutrients in around the edges when you feel too full to eat a complete meal.

6 cups vegetable broth

2 (14-ounce) cans kidney beans, rinsed and drained

1 (14-ounce) can diced tomatoes

2 carrots, diced

1 zucchini, diced

1 small onion, diced

1 tablespoon fresh lemon juice

½ teaspoon salt

½ teaspoon garlic powder

½ teaspoon dried oregano

½ teaspoon dried basil

1 cup chopped fresh spinach

1. In a large stockpot, combine the broth, beans, tomatoes and their juices, carrot, zucchini, onion, lemon juice, salt, garlic powder, oregano, and basil.

2. Cover, bring to a boil, reduce the heat to medium low, and simmer for 10 minutes.

3. Stir in the spinach and let wilt for about 5 minutes before serving.

Ingredient tip: If you're not vegetarian, replace the vegetable broth with protein-packed and glycine-rich bone broth. If using a low-sodium broth, more seasoning may be desired.

Per serving: Calories: 332; Total Fat: 3g; Saturated Fat: 1g; Cholesterol: 0mg; Sodium: 910mg; Carbohydrates: 53g; Fiber: 16g; Protein: 25g

Walnut Tacos

GLUTEN-FREE, VEGETARIAN

SERVES 6

PREP TIME: 30 minutes / **COOK TIME:** 40 minutes

Think tacos need to be made with meat to be satisfying? Think again. These tacos give this dish a boost of plant-based proteins, healthy fats, and fiber to support a healthy pregnancy. Even if you are a carnivore, you will enjoy this recipe when taco night rolls around.

1 cup cauliflower, chopped

2 tablespoons extra-virgin olive oil, divided

1 cup chopped onion

½ cup chopped red bell pepper

1 garlic clove, minced

1 jalapeño, minced

½ cup vegetable broth

¼ cup tomato paste

2 teaspoons chili powder

1 cup walnuts, chopped

12 corn tortillas, warmed

1½ cups shredded iceberg lettuce

¾ cup shredded white cheddar cheese

Lime wedges, for serving

1. Preheat the oven to 450°F.

2. On a baking sheet, drizzle the cauliflower with 1 tablespoon of olive oil in a single layer and roast for 25 minutes.

3. In a large skillet, heat the remaining tablespoon of olive oil over medium heat. Add the onion and bell pepper and sauté for 5 minutes until softened.

4. Add the jalapeño and garlic and cook for 2 more minutes. Stir in the broth, tomato paste, and chili powder. Cook until the mixture is thick and the excess broth has cooked off. Stir in the cauliflower mixture and walnuts.

5. Spoon the mixture into warmed tortillas and top with lettuce, cheese, and a squeeze of fresh lime.

Substitution tip: Swap the walnuts with pistachios for an equally nutritious meat-free taco. Feel free to include any spices that you love—cumin and cilantro are wonderful additions.

Per serving: Calories: 369; Total Fat: 24g; Saturated Fat: 5g; Cholesterol: 14mg; Sodium: 203mg; Carbohydrates: 34g; Fiber: 6g; Protein: 11g

Chicken with Dates

DAIRY-FREE, NUT-FREE

SERVES 4

PREP TIME: 30 minutes / **COOK TIME:** 1 hour

This chicken recipe is naturally sweetened with dates, a fruit that, when consumed during the last 4 weeks of pregnancy, has been shown to possibly result in a lower C-section rate and less need for certain medications during labor. The natural fiber found in these wrinkly fruits can help keep the bowel movements, well, moving. Because constipation is a symptom some people experience in late pregnancy, loading up on fiber can be very helpful to keep the bowels healthy. Serve over quinoa for even more fiber.

8 bone-in, skin-on chicken thighs

¼ teaspoon freshly ground black pepper

¼ teaspoon salt

2 tablespoons extra-virgin olive oil, divided

3 cups diced yellow onion

1 tablespoon minced fresh ginger

2 tablespoons all-purpose flour

1½ teaspoons ground cinnamon

½ teaspoon ground cumin

½ teaspoon paprika

2 cups reduced-sodium chicken broth

½ cup whole pitted dates, chopped

3 tablespoons fresh lemon juice

¼ cup fresh basil leaves

1. Sprinkle the chicken with pepper and salt.

2. In a 10-quart Dutch oven or heavy pot, heat 1 tablespoon of olive oil over medium heat. Add the chicken thighs, skin-side down, to the pan. Cook for 5 minutes on each side or until browned. Transfer the chicken to a plate and set aside.

3. In the same Dutch oven, heat the remaining tablespoon of olive oil over medium heat, and add the onion and ginger. Sauté for 10 minutes, or until the onion becomes translucent.

4. Stir in the flour, cinnamon, cumin, and paprika, then add the broth. Bring to a boil for 3 minutes, stirring occasionally.

5. Arrange the cooked chicken over the sauce in the pan. Cover, reduce the heat to low, and cook for 12 minutes.

6. Stir in the dates. Simmer for 10 minutes, or until chicken is cooked through.

7. Stir in the lemon juice. Transfer the chicken to a serving dish and top with sauce. Garnish with basil leaves.

Substitution tip: You can easily substitute dried apricots or prunes for the dates, and this dish will still taste great. Just keep in mind that the data surrounding the benefits of eating dates during pregnancy does not also apply to these fruit alternatives.

Per serving: Calories: 683; Total Fat: 45g; Saturated Fat: 11g; Cholesterol: 220mg; Sodium: 621mg; Carbohydrates: 34g; Fiber: 5g; Protein: 42g

Mediterranean-Inspired Sheet Pan Chicken

GLUTEN-FREE, NUT-FREE

SERVES 6

PREP TIME: 5 minutes, plus 30 minutes chill time / **COOK TIME:** 25 minutes

Olives are a sneaky source of non-heme iron and fiber in a small package. But their main claim to fame is their high monounsaturated–fatty acid content, which has been shown to reduce the risk of cardiovascular disease and reduce blood pressure. They also offer a diverse range of anti-inflammatory and antioxidant nutrients that benefit pregnancy.

1 large egg

2 tablespoons fresh lemon juice

3 garlic cloves, minced

¾ teaspoon salt, divided

4 boneless chicken breasts

1 cup grated Parmesan cheese

2 cups chopped cauliflower

2 cups chopped green beans

1 cup cherry tomatoes

1 cup mixed olives, pitted

2 tablespoons ghee, melted

Freshly ground black pepper

1. Preheat the oven to 400°F. Line a baking pan with parchment paper.

2. In a large bowl, whisk together the egg, lemon juice, garlic, and ½ teaspoon of salt. Add each chicken breast into the bowl with the egg mixture, turning to make sure it's covered with the egg. Cover the bowl and refrigerate for 30 minutes.

3. Place the chicken on the baking sheet and sprinkle with the Parmesan.

4. In a large bowl, combine the cauliflower, green beans, tomatoes, olives, ghee, pepper, and the remaining ¼ teaspoon of salt. Stir well to coat. Spoon the vegetables around the chicken in the baking pan.

5. Bake for 25 minutes, stirring and flipping the ingredients halfway through, until the juices run clear.

6. Spoon onto plates and serve hot.

Cooking tip: Avoid aluminum baking sheets and aluminum foil when cooking. There is no studied use for aluminum in the body, and it is a toxin that can easily leach into your food.

Per serving: Calories: 273; Total Fat: 17g; Saturated Fat: 6g; Cholesterol: 51mg; Sodium: 488mg; Carbohydrates: 7g; Fiber: 3g; Protein: 26g

Ground Turkey and Butternut Squash Chili

DAIRY-FREE, GLUTEN-FREE, NUT-FREE, FREEZER-FRIENDLY

SERVES 6

PREP TIME: 15 minutes / **COOK TIME:** 25 minutes

Hearty butternut squash is easy to cook and digest. When combined with the healthy fats from the turkey, the beta-carotene (preformed vitamin A) in the squash is even better absorbed by your body. If using store-bought broth, be aware of the potentially higher sodium content and consider not adding any more salt.

1 pound ground turkey

1 medium red onion, chopped

1 red bell pepper, chopped

2 cups diced butternut squash

1 cup frozen sweet corn

1 (28-ounce) can diced tomatoes

2 cups Slow Cooker Beef Bone Broth (page 87) or store-bought

1 (15-ounce) can black beans, rinsed and drained

1 tablespoon chili powder

1 teaspoon garlic powder

1 teaspoon ground cumin

½ teaspoon salt

¼ teaspoon ground cinnamon

1. In a 4- to 6-quart stockpot, cook the turkey over medium heat for about 5 minutes, using a spoon to break it up as it browns.

2. Push the turkey to the sides of the pot and add the onion and bell pepper to the center. Cook for about 3 minutes, until they start to soften. Add the squash and corn and cook for another 3 to 5 minutes.

3. Add the tomatoes and their juices, broth, beans, chili powder, garlic powder, cumin, salt, and cinnamon. Cover and cook on low for 10 minutes, stirring occasionally, until the flavors meld.

4. Serve with optional toppings like whole-milk yogurt, sliced scallions or radishes, or chopped cilantro.

Time-Saving tip: To speed up this recipe, purchase organic prechopped frozen veggies in place of the bell pepper and butternut squash.

Per serving: Calories: 275; Total Fat: 3g; Saturated Fat: 1g; Cholesterol: 41mg; Sodium: 271mg; Carbohydrates: 34g; Fiber: 9g; Protein: 32g

Tomato and Feta Baked Cod

GLUTEN-FREE, NUT-FREE

SERVES 4

PREP TIME: 10 minutes / **COOK TIME:** 25 minutes

....

Cod is a versatile fish that fuels your pregnant body with a slew of important nutrients like DHA and iodine to support baby's brain development. Enjoy this simple dinner that checks plenty of pregnancy-friendly food boxes. The sprinkle of feta on top gives this dish a boost of bone-building calcium along with some unique flavor.

....

2 cups new potatoes, quartered

¼ cup extra-virgin olive oil, divided

2 garlic cloves, minced

2 cups cherry tomatoes

4 (4-ounce) cod fillets

2 tablespoons chopped fresh parsley

Salt

Freshly ground black pepper

½ cup pasteurized feta cheese

1 lemon, quartered

1. Preheat the oven to 400°F.

2. On a baking sheet, toss the potatoes with 2 tablespoons of olive oil and the garlic. Spread the potatoes out in a single layer and roast for 15 minutes.

3. Add the tomatoes, cod, and parsley to the pan. Drizzle with the remaining 2 tablespoons of olive oil and season with salt and pepper to taste.

4. Bake for 10 minutes until cooked through.

5. Sprinkle the feta cheese on top and garnish with lemon wedges.

Cooking tip: If you know you are going to want dinner on the table ASAP, pre-roast the potatoes and heat them up before you enjoy your meal. If cod is not available, use pollock instead.

....

Per serving: Calories: 354; Total Fat: 21g; Saturated Fat: 6g; Cholesterol: 86mg; Sodium: 740mg; Carbohydrates: 21g; Fiber: 2g; Protein: 26g

Pan-Fried Lemon Butter Trout

GLUTEN-FREE, NUT-FREE

SERVES 2

PREP TIME: 5 minutes / **COOK TIME:** 10 minutes

Trout is an excellent and yummy way to get more vitamin D and B_{12} into your third-trimester diet, aiding in sustained energy and immunity as you power through to the end. Pair this with a whole grain and steamed veggies or a green salad for a complete meal.

1 teaspoon, plus 2 tablespoons ghee or
  grass-fed butter

2 (4-ounce) trout fillets

¼ cup fresh lemon juice

¼ teaspoon salt

Freshly ground black pepper

1 lemon, thinly sliced

1. In a large skillet, melt 1 teaspoon of ghee over medium heat. Add the trout fillets and cook for 3 minutes on each side, until the center is flaky. Transfer to two plates.

2. In the same skillet, mix together the lemon juice, salt, and pepper and bring to a simmer. Add the remaining 2 tablespoons of ghee and whisk together well.

3. Spoon the sauce over the fish and garnish with lemon slices before serving.

Ingredient tip: Capers or caramelized onions complement this dish well.

Per serving: Calories: 271; Total Fat: 14g; Saturated Fat: 5g; Cholesterol: 115mg; Sodium: 285mg; Carbohydrates: 1g; Fiber: 0g; Protein: 34g

Spaghetti with Sardines and Greens

DAIRY-FREE, GLUTEN-FREE, NUT-FREE

SERVES 4

PREP TIME: 10 minutes / **COOK TIME:** 20 minutes

Believe it or not, this dairy-free dish is filled with calcium, vitamin D, and omega-3s. The sardines are the secret ingredient—they are an excellent source of all three nutrients, plus protein and a massive amount of vitamin B_{12}.

8 ounces chickpea pasta

1 tablespoon extra-virgin olive oil

2 (4.4-ounce) cans oil-packed sardines, chopped into 1-inch pieces, oil reserved

2 teaspoons Dijon mustard

¾ cup diced zucchini

½ teaspoon garlic powder

¼ cup water

2 cups baby arugula

⅓ cup sliced green olives

2 tablespoons capers (optional)

1 tablespoon fresh lemon juice

1. Bring a large pot of water to a boil and cook the pasta according to the package directions. Drain and drizzle with the olive oil. Set aside.

2. In a cast-iron skillet, heat 1 tablespoon of the reserved sardine oil over medium heat. Add the sardines and mustard and cook for about 2 minutes until heated through. Transfer to a plate.

3. In the same skillet, mix together the zucchini and garlic powder and cook for 2 to 3 minutes, stirring to combine. Add the pasta and water and cook for 2 minutes until heated through.

4. Add the arugula, olives, and capers (if using) and simmer over low heat for 2 minutes. Stir in the lemon juice and sardines and serve warm.

Ingredient tip: The small, savory capers we consume in many Mediterranean dishes are the small flower buds of the caper bush. These are typically eaten after being pickled.

Per serving: Calories: 394; Total Fat: 21g; Saturated Fat: 6g; Cholesterol: 15mg; Sodium: 547mg; Carbohydrates: 35g; Fiber: 9g; Protein: 16g

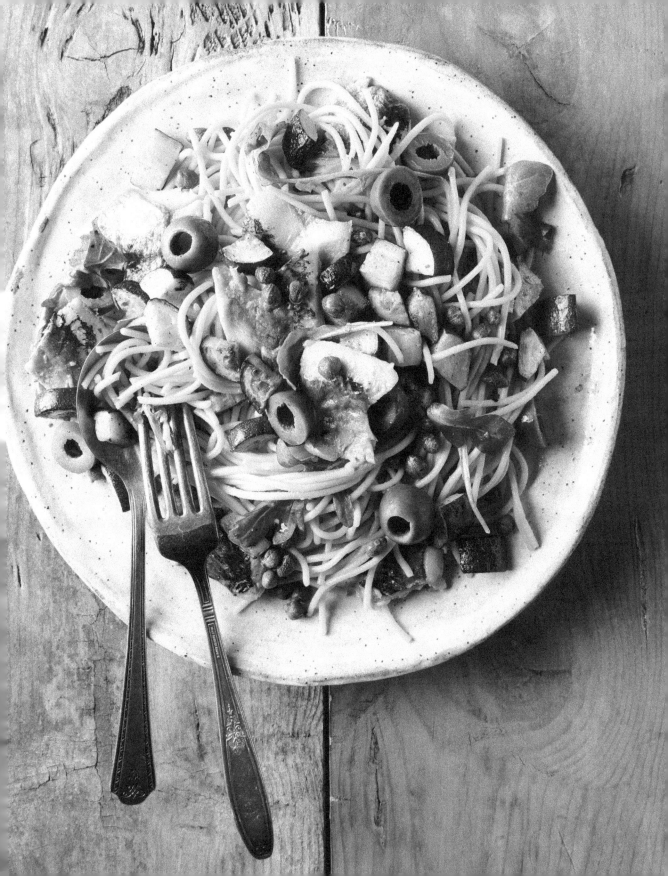

Slow Cooker Short Ribs

GLUTEN-FREE, NUT-FREE

SERVES 6

PREP TIME: 15 minutes / **COOK TIME:** 6 to 8 hours

Slow-cooked meat is a vital source of nutrition for pregnant mamas. Not only is it a complete protein, but it's densely packed with minerals, B vitamins, and the most readily absorbed forms of both iron and zinc. This recipe is also rich in the amino acid glycine, necessary for baby's DNA synthesis and collagen creation.

3 pounds bone-in short ribs

½ teaspoon salt

Freshly ground black pepper

3 tablespoons butter

2 cups Slow Cooker Beef Bone Broth (page 87) or store-bought

1 medium yellow onion, chopped

8 tablespoons coconut aminos

1 teaspoon fresh lemon juice

1 teaspoon garlic powder

1 teaspoon onion powder

½ teaspoon dried rosemary

1. Season the ribs with the salt and pepper.

2. In a large cast-iron skillet, melt the butter over high heat. Add the ribs and sear on each side for 1 minute.

3. In a slow cooker, mix together the broth, onion, coconut aminos, lemon juice, garlic powder, onion powder, and rosemary. Add the ribs and drizzle any remaining butter on top. Cook on low for 6 to 8 hours, until the meat is falling-off-the-bone tender.

Ingredient tip: Serve these ribs alongside a buttery veggie mash, made with potato, cauliflower, and romanesco, for an extra special treat. Garnish with parsley and dill.

Per serving: Calories: 552; Total Fat: 44g; Saturated Fat: 21g; Cholesterol: 195mg; Sodium: 418mg; Carbohydrates: 4g; Fiber: 1g; Protein: 39g

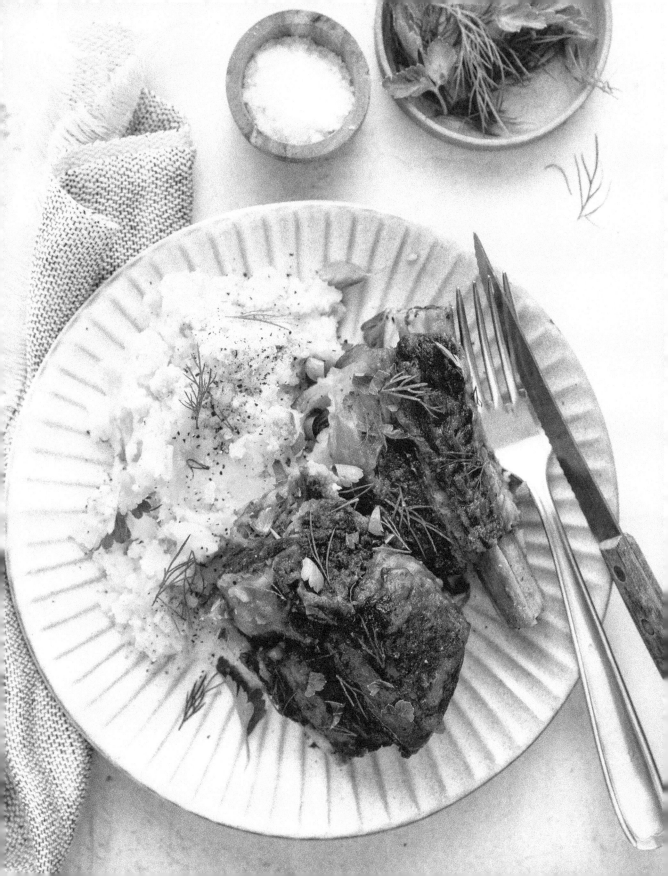

Grilled Beef Kabobs with Brown Rice

DAIRY-FREE, NUT-FREE

SERVES 4

PREP TIME: 20 minutes / **COOK TIME:** 8 minutes

In the second and third trimester, iron needs increase. Beef is an excellent source of iron and a high-quality protein to support baby's growing body, along with zinc to support a healthy immune system.

⅓ cup low-sodium soy sauce

3 tablespoons pineapple juice

2 tablespoons extra-virgin olive oil

2 tablespoons apple cider vinegar

1 teaspoon freshly ground black pepper

1 pound boneless top sirloin steak, cut into cubes

1 red bell pepper, cut into 2-inch squares

1 zucchini, cut into 2-inch squares

1 red onion, cut into 2-inch squares

8 button mushrooms

2 cups cooked brown rice

1. In a medium bowl, whisk the soy sauce, pineapple juice, olive oil, vinegar, and black pepper together. Add the steak to the bowl and mix together. Marinate for at least 15 minutes.

2. Preheat the grill to high heat.

3. Thread the marinated steak onto skewers, alternating between the meat, bell pepper, zucchini, onion, and mushroom. Leave a little bit of space between the pieces so they can cook evenly on the grill.

4. Brush a little remaining marinade onto the meat and veggies.

5. Grill the kabobs for 8 to 10 minutes, turning every couple of minutes, until cooked through.

6. Serve over brown rice.

Cooking tip: A grill pan can be used on the stovetop to cook the kabobs if a grill is not available. Chicken can be used if beef is being avoided. For a sweet addition, include fresh pineapple pieces on the kebab before grilling.

Per serving: Calories: 390; Total Fat: 13g; Saturated Fat: 3g; Cholesterol: 60mg; Sodium: 837mg; Carbohydrates: 36g; Fiber: 4g; Protein: 33g

Homemade Granola Bars

DAIRY-FREE, VEGETARIAN, FREEZER-FRIENDLY

SERVES 6

PREP TIME: 10 minutes / **COOK TIME:** 10 minutes

Store-bought granola bars are convenient, but they can be loaded with sugar and fillers. Making your own granola bars is surprisingly easy and even tastier than the prepackaged varieties. Including dates and maple syrup adds some natural sweetness and antioxidants.

1½ cups old-fashioned rolled oats

1 cup unsalted almonds, chopped

1 heaping packed cup pitted dates

½ cup dried golden raisins

¼ cup pure maple syrup

¼ cup creamy salted natural peanut butter or almond butter

1. Preheat the oven to 350°F.

2. On a baking sheet, toast the oats and almonds in oven for 10 minutes.

3. In a food processor, blend the dates until they reach a dough-like consistency, about 1 minute.

4. In a large mixing bowl, combine the oats, almonds, dates, and raisins.

5. In a small saucepan, warm the maple syrup and peanut butter over low heat. Stir until well combined. Pour the maple and peanut butter mixture over the oat mixture and mix well.

6. Line an 8-inch square baking dish with plastic wrap or parchment paper. Press the mixture into the prepared baking dish until flattened.

7. Cover with plastic wrap, and place in the freezer for 10 minutes.

8. Cut into bars and remove from the pan. Store in an airtight container for 3 days.

Time-Saving tip: Make an extra batch of granola bars and freeze them to enjoy during your busy postpartum weeks. Better yet, pack some in your overnight hospital bag to enjoy during your hospital stay.

Per serving: Calories: 408; Total Fat: 19g; Saturated Fat: 2g; Cholesterol: 0mg; Sodium: 51mg; Carbohydrates: 57g; Fiber: 7g; Protein: 10g

Nutty Energy Bites

DAIRY-FREE, VEGETARIAN

SERVES 6

PREP TIME: 10 minutes, plus 20 minutes to chill

Three tablespoons of hemp hearts contain around 14 grams of total fat, 11 grams of protein, and only 2 grams of carbohydrates. That's a fantastic macronutrient profile! These tiny seeds are also an excellent source of iron, zinc, and magnesium, not to mention a good amount of potassium to help balance out any excess sodium and support healthy blood pressure. I've also included Brazil nuts for their super protective selenium content. They don't call them energy bites for nothing!

1 cup Brazil nuts

½ cup hemp hearts

8 pitted Medjool dates

½ cup rolled oats

1 tablespoon ground flaxseed

1 tablespoon almond butter

1 tablespoon coconut oil

1 teaspoon pure vanilla extract or vanilla bean powder

½ teaspoon ground cinnamon

Dash salt

1. In a food processor, pulse the Brazil nuts and hemp hearts until finely ground. Add the dates and oats slowly and continue to pulse. Add the flaxseed, almond butter, coconut oil, vanilla, cinnamon, and salt and continue to process until the mixture starts to ball up in the food processor.

2. Using a spoon, scoop out about a tablespoon of the mixture and use your hands to form a ball. Place it on a plate and repeat with the rest of the mixture.

3. Cover with plastic wrap and place in the refrigerator for at least 20 minutes before serving. Store in an airtight container in the refrigerator for up to 6 days.

Cooking tip: If the mixture feels too dry and crumbly, add 1 to 2 tablespoons of water and pulse a few more times before forming the balls. I also love to add 2 tablespoons of chocolate chips. I like Enjoy Life brand because it's allergen-friendly and soy-free.

Per serving: Calories: 380; Total Fat: 25g; Saturated Fat: 6g; Cholesterol: 0mg; Sodium: 40mg; Carbohydrates: 34g; Fiber: 6g; Protein: 10g

Crispy Chili Chickpeas

DAIRY-FREE, GLUTEN-FREE, NUT-FREE, VEGETARIAN

MAKES 2 CUPS

PREP TIME: 5 minutes / **COOK TIME:** 20 minutes

Chickpeas are packed with phytonutrients that possess powerful anti-inflammatory nutrients, not to mention a healthy dose of non-heme iron and zinc. To keep this snack in regular rotation, try mixing in different spices, such as cumin, garlic powder, or paprika, so you won't get bored.

4 cups canned chickpeas, rinsed, and dried with paper towels

2 tablespoons extra-virgin olive oil

1 teaspoon chili powder

¾ teaspoon salt

1. Preheat the oven to 400°F. Line a baking pan with parchment paper.

2. Spread the chickpeas in the baking pan in one layer and coat them with the olive oil.

3. Bake for 20 minutes, stirring halfway through, until crisp.

4. Toss with the chili powder and salt and serve.

Per serving (½ cup): Calories: 166; Total Fat: 6g; Saturated Fat: 1g; Cholesterol: 0mg; Sodium: 188mg; Carbohydrates: 23g; Fiber: 6g; Protein: 7g

Nuts for Dates

DAIRY-FREE, GLUTEN-FREE, VEGETARIAN

SERVES 6

PREP TIME: 10 minutes

....

Dates, while high in natural sugar, possess an innate ability to support you in labor. As long as you balance their sugar with healthy fats and protein, like in this recipe, dates can be the perfect snack toward the end of your pregnancy. I chose Brazil nuts for their perfect size here, but also because they act as a supplement in terms of their wonderful selenium content.

....

12 Medjool dates, pitted

¼ cup peanut butter

12 Brazil nuts

1. Cut open each date. Using a small spatula, spread a teaspoon of peanut butter inside.

2. Insert a Brazil nut into each, then close the date back up.

3. Store in an airtight container in the refrigerator for up to 1 week.

Ingredient tip: While exposing baby to potential allergens (like peanuts) in utero is proven to be helpful down the line, if you already know you have an adverse reaction to peanuts, swap in almond or cashew butter here.

....

Per serving (2 dates): Calories: 263; Total Fat: 12g; Saturated Fat: 3g; Cholesterol: 0mg; Sodium: 49mg; Carbohydrates: 40g; Fiber: 5g; Protein: 5g

Frozen Yogurt Bark

GLUTEN-FREE, NUT-FREE, VEGETARIAN, FREEZER-FRIENDLY

SERVES 6

PREP TIME: 2 minutes, plus 3 hours to chill

Frozen yogurt bark is packed with bone-supporting nutrients like calcium and satisfies the sweet tooth. Using fruit instead of sugar to sweeten this recipe helps fuel your body with nutrients like vitamin C and folate. Fun fact: The live probiotics found in yogurt become dormant when they are frozen. Once they reach the warmth of your stomach, the probiotics become active again and can colonize your gut and help keep it healthy. Combining probiotics with prebiotic foods (undigestible starch that probiotics use as fuel) helps ensure the probiotics remain healthy and can perform health benefits. Prebiotic-rich foods include berries, underripe bananas, and chicory root.

2 cups plain whole milk yogurt

½ cup blueberries

1 teaspoon pure maple syrup

¼ cup hemp seeds

1. Line a baking sheet with wax paper.

2. In a blender, blend the yogurt, blueberries, and maple syrup.

3. Spread the mixture evenly onto the wax paper. Sprinkle with the hemp seeds and freeze until solid, about 3 hours.

4. Alternatively, sprinkle the blueberries on top of the yogurt mixture just before freezing.

Storage tip: Once frozen, break the yogurt into chunks and transfer to a freezer bag.

Per serving: Calories: 105; Total Fat: 6g; Saturated Fat: 2g; Cholesterol: 11mg; Sodium: 38mg; Carbohydrates: 7g; Fiber: 1g; Protein: 5g

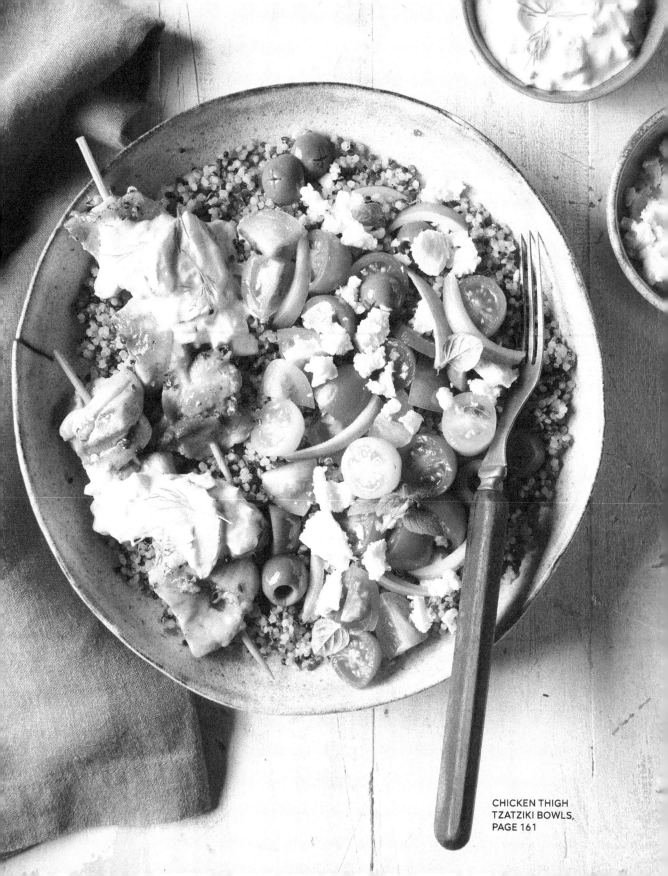

CHICKEN THIGH
TZATZIKI BOWLS,
PAGE 161

While you're pregnant, there is nutrition information coming from 100 different directions. Once baby is born and you heal from delivery and at the same time produce enough milk to keep the new baby nourished (if you are breastfeeding), advice gets a little more lean, especially from health care providers. Unfortunately, the nutrition advice you'll get when breastfeeding may not go beyond "keep taking a prenatal vitamin."

In this chapter, you'll learn how you should eat to support your healing from birth—regardless of whether you had your baby vaginally or via C-section—and how to eat to support your breastfeeding journey if you are nursing.

Postpartum Healing

Giving birth is no easy feat. If you delivered your baby vaginally, you may have exerted yourself by going through labor. Additionally, you may have experienced blood loss and electrolyte loss, both of which can be improved with proper nutrition. Some people experience tearing or require surgery during delivery, in which case supporting healthy skin repair by eating the right foods can be a positive effort.

Iron

If you experienced blood loss, it is important to take in iron to rebuild your blood count. It is not recommended to take iron supplements unless advised by your doctor, because these pills may be constipating. Focus on food sources of iron: beef, chicken, and seafood for heme sources, and legumes, leafy greens, and seeds for non-heme sources. If choosing non-heme iron sources, eat them with a boost of vitamin C to maximize absorption—think kiwi, oranges, and strawberries. Foods like certain oats and cereals are fortified with iron and are convenient options.

Protein, Amino Acids, and Micronutrients

You just carried a baby for nine months. Naturally, your skin stretched and changed. No matter how you delivered your baby, it is likely in need of some healing. Certain amino acids are thought to offer more skin support than others. Glycine and proline are two key amino acids that should be a focus during the fourth trimester. Foods like bone broth, chicken with skin, and legumes will fuel your body with key amino acids. Some people lean on collagen peptides to support their skin as well, although there is very little evidence in the medical literature that suggests that this product plays a direct role on postpartum skin support.

Protein helps with the rebuilding and regrowth that your body may need. Foods like eggs, meats, and tofu are all excellent protein sources. Micronutrients that may help support your skin postpartum include zinc (from meats, whole grains, and oysters) and vitamin C (from citrus, red bell pepper, and tomatoes).

Fiber

Moving your bowels can be a real challenge after your baby is born. Stay ahead of the constipation and make a point to eat 25 to 35 grams of fiber per day, along with drinking a lot of water. Foods like fruit with the skin still on, grains, vegetables, and chia seeds can help you stay regular.

WHAT TO EXPECT THIS TRIMESTER

How Baby Is Developing: Your baby is adjusting to a world outside the womb. Imagine going from a cozy, dark, and warm place to the world as we know it—strange noises, bright lights, and different smells. Baby may be cranky and snuggly at times, and it is a time for a lot of nurturing.

Changes in Mom: The first three months postpartum is also a time you need to focus on yourself. As challenging as it may sound, caring for yourself needs to be on the top of the priority list. Post-birth requires healing, and proper nutrition will help support your energy levels when you are sleeping in three-hour increments.

Foods to Enjoy: Brazil nuts, eggs, red meat, carrots, oats, almonds, chia seeds, and salmon.

Nutrition Needs for Nursing

If you are feeding your baby with breastmilk, your baby will be getting a slew of benefits regardless of what you are eating. However, there are some nutrients that are found in breastmilk that are dependent on mom's intake and therefore should be a focus. Most health care providers recommend that lactating people continue to take a prenatal vitamin. Many of the following nutrients are also important for recovery in general, even if you're not breastfeeding. Some parents call this process breastfeeding, others call it chestfeeding or nursing, but I'll be using the common phrase *breastfeeding*.

Calories

Thanks to celebrities in the media, many people believe that it is possible to be "bikini ready" days after giving birth. Not only is it unsafe to start exercising and restricting calories shortly after delivery, it's also unrealistic. Calories are needed for healing, for lactation support, and to help you have the energy you need to care for your new baby.

According to the National Institutes of Health, lactating people need an additional 450 to 500 calories per day. Nursing moms also need about 65 grams of protein per day, according to the Dietary Guidelines for Americans. Choosing protein sources rich in the amino acid glycine may also support the healing process. Think foods that incorporate connective tissue like skin-on or stew meats.

Protein

Having quick protein-rich snacks that are easy to eat with one hand will help you meet your needs. Hard-boiled eggs are a great grab-and-go snack. A nut butter and fruit combo (like fresh apple and almond butter) is also an easy no-prep snack.

Choline-Rich Foods

Choline is needed in higher amounts when mom is lactating, because this nutrient is key to brain development for your baby and is transferred through breastmilk. Many infant formulas are supplemented with this nutrient, and breastmilk may provide adequate amounts if mom takes in enough. Although your needs have increased to 550mg/day, some studies suggest that baby benefits from even more than that!

One of the best sources of choline is egg yolks. Experts recommend including a choline supplement into their regimen because there are only so many egg yolks a person can eat in a day, and most generic prenatal vitamins provide a very small amount of this nutrient. If you are eliminating eggs from your diet, you absolutely should consider a choline supplement to support your baby's brain development during this critical time. Other food sources of choline include liver, peanuts, and cauliflower.

DHA

DHA is an omega-3 fatty acid that is essential for brain and vision development for baby. The American Academy of Pediatrics recommends that breastfeeding mothers take in 200 to 300mg of omega-3 fatty acids per day. Adequate DHA may benefit mom as well. Experts suggest that taking in adequate amounts may protect against postpartum depression symptoms and promote over-all wellness.

Choosing two servings of low-mercury seafood (like salmon or shrimp) can help you meet your goals. Even if your prenatal vitamin has DHA in it, eating fish and seafood is still recommended to get all the benefits that can't be bottled up in pill form.

Selenium-Rich Foods

Selenium has a role as an antioxidant, in thyroid hormone metabolism, and in immune function. Levels of selenium in breast milk are dependent on mom's intake. If you are already taking in two servings of low-mercury foods, you are on the right track for getting enough selenium (because many fish choices are rich in selenium). If not, and if your prenatal vitamin doesn't include selenium, eating one Brazil nut every other day is a great way to naturally get a boost of this nutrient.

Iodine

Iodine is important for your new baby's health, specifically for thyroid function and proper brain development. It's also an important nutrient for you, because taking in adequate amounts may reduce the risk of developing postpartum thyroid dysfunction and also supports breast health.

Lactating mom's iodine needs are higher than they were during pregnancy according to the National Institutes of Health, and one easy way to incorporate more iodine is to choose salt that has been fortified with this nutrient. Seafood, eggs, dairy, and seaweed are other good iodine-rich choices.

Vitamin D

Vitamin D is essential to baby to prevent a condition called rickets as well as other health concerns. Many doctors recommend breastfed babies receive vitamin D supplementation of 400 IU/day, but that does not mean that mom is off the hook with getting enough of this nutrient, too. Enough vitamin D intake will support mom's bone health and overall well-being. Some studies suggest that baby wouldn't need to be supplemented if mom takes in 6,400 IU of vitamin D per day through her own supplementation, but this option should not be explored without a doctor's guidance.

Vitamin A

Vitamin A is critical to a new baby's development during lactation. Vitamin A is one key nutrient that levels are influenced by mom's intake. Among other roles, vitamin A supports baby's immune system. Colostrum is especially high in this vitamin and is the reason why it has that yellowish tinge to it.

Examples of foods rich in the natural beta-carotene form of vitamin A are often naturally orange in color like sweet potatoes and cantaloupe. Foods rich in beta-carotene are a safe bet when lactating. However, a little bit of preformed vitamin A (found mostly in animal and dairy fats) is needed, too.

Calcium

Some studies have shown a 3 to 5 percent reduction in a mother's bone mass while they are breastfeeding, most likely due to an insufficient amount of calcium in their diet. If mom's diet is lacking in calcium, their bodies will take calcium from their bones to supply it to the nursing infant.

To protect themselves from bone loss during lactation, almost all mothers need to take 1,000mg of calcium per day. It is entirely possible to eat enough foods that contain calcium even when you are eliminating milk proteins from your diet. Milk substitutes are fortified with calcium, as are nondairy yogurts and some orange juices. Many fruits and veggies are natural sources of calcium, too. Be mindful not to supplement with more than 500mg at a time, and to avoid taking calcium supplements at the same time that you supplement with iron (both minerals compete for absorption).

Water

Contrary to Dr. Google, drinking more water will not increase your milk supply. However, staying hydrated is very important when breastfeeding. The act of producing breastmilk uses a lot of water, and replenishing will keep mom feeling energized and healthy. The postpartum/lactation stage is a beautiful time, but it can be exhausting and difficult to prioritize your nutrition.

A pregnant person's self-care should be emphasized to make sure they are able to give baby everything they need emotionally and nutritionally. Using these tips and leaning on your own "village" is key.

Ask for help when you need it. New moms may feel pressure to "do it all," and do it well. While new mothers are incredible, they're not superhuman—especially on limited sleep. If you need help caring for your baby, don't wait for somebody to offer. It takes a strong person to recognize when they need a hand and to seek it out. If you know that you need help but don't know where to begin, your health care provider is a good starting place to explore your options.

Set up a breastfeeding station stocked with supplies. Set up a nursing station stacked with the essentials, including nipple cream, burp clothes, diapers, hair ties, and snacks for mom. Anything that you may need should be on that cart.

Have a postpartum care kit handy. Having the right supplies for your own care is extremely necessary. Stool softeners, a peri bottle (if you had a vaginal delivery), and nursing bras are all must-haves.

Know your limits and say "no" when needed. If your cousin wants to come over to see the baby but you're so tired that you're seeing double, don't prioritize their feelings over your own needs. Saying no to visits, commitments, and, well, anything is okay these days. You need to do what is good for you, because ultimately, what is good for you is good for your baby, too.

About the Postpartum Meal Plans

Having a new baby in tow can make meal planning a challenge. Some days can get so busy that a new parent can quite possibly completely forget to eat! These meal plan suggestions are rich in nutrient-dense foods that are simple to prepare and can often be enjoyed with one hand (because your other hand is likely occupied holding your little one). While these plans are focused on the breastfeeding mother, they are completely appropriate for the formula-feeding parent as well.

Month 10 Sample Meal Plan

	BREAKFAST	LUNCH	DINNER	SNACK/ DESSERT
DAY 1	Chia-Berry Overnight Oats (page 149)	Quinoa and red bean salad (scallions, shredded carrot, pumpkin seeds, golden raisins, kidney beans, quinoa, avocado oil, and apple cider vinegar) with 1 apple	Slow Cooker Chicken with Mango Salsa (page 162) with ½ cup brown rice	Rice cakes topped with avocado and chopped egg
DAY 2	Breakfast Sandwich (page 152) with ½ cup fruit salad	Leftover Slow Cooker Chicken with Mango Salsa with rice	Scallop and Strawberry Salad (page 153)	2 Lactation Cookies (page 165) and glass of milk or nondairy alternative
DAY 3	Leftover Chia-Berry Overnight Oats	Leftover Scallop and Strawberry Salad	Warming Sausage Soup (page 155)	Broiled Grapefruit with Frozen Yogurt and Crushed Brazil Nuts (page 166)
DAY 4	Leftover Breakfast Sandwich with ½ cup fruit salad	Leftover Warming Sausage Soup with ½ cup berries	Zucchini Noodles with Burst Cherry Tomatoes and Garlic (page 160)	Cucumber slices with dill-avocado dip (½ tablespoons dill, ½ avocado, ½ tablespoon mayonnaise, ¼ lemon, ½ teaspoon minced garlic, and ¼ teaspoon dried oregano)
DAY 5	Leftover Breakfast Sandwich with ½ cup fruit salad	Leftover Zucchini Noodles with Burst Cherry Tomatoes and Garlic	Winter Lentil Stew (page 158)	Leftover Broiled Grapefruit with Frozen Yogurt and Crushed Brazil Nuts
DAY 6	Scrambled eggs with Swiss cheese, spinach, and roasted sweet potato cubes with a sliced orange	Leftover Winter Lentil Stew	Brisket with Prunes and Sweet Potatoes (page 164)	2 leftover Lactation Cookies and glass of milk or nondairy alternative
DAY 7	Quinoa Breakie Bowl (page 151)	Lemon, Arugula, and Quinoa Salad (page 154)	Leftover Brisket with Prunes and Sweet Potatoes	Milk-Boosting Granola (page 168)

Month 11 Sample Meal Plan

	BREAKFAST	LUNCH	DINNER	SNACK/DESSERT
DAY 1	Milk-Boosting Granola (page 168) with ½ cup reduced-fat Greek yogurt and fresh berries	Wrap with 3 ounces turkey, avocado, and nitrite-free bacon with 1 orange and 1 square dark chocolate	Chicken Thigh Tzatziki Bowls (page 161)	Broiled Grapefruit with Frozen Yogurt and Crushed Brazil Nuts (page 166)
DAY 2	Leftover Milk-Boosting Granola with ½ cup reduced-fat Greek yogurt and fresh berries	Leftover Chicken Thigh Tzatziki Bowls	Bone Broth Ramen (page 159) with 8 strawberries	2 Lactation Cookies (page 165) with a glass of reduced-fat milk or nondairy alternative
DAY 3	Creamiest Caramel Steel-Cut Oats (page 150)	Leftover Bone Broth Ramen and ½ cup blueberries	Lemon-Garlic Salmon and Asparagus (page 163)	Leftover Broiled Grapefruit with Frozen Yogurt and Crushed Brazil Nuts
DAY 4	Cinnamon, applesauce, and cottage cheese parfait topped with leftover Milk-Boosting Granola	Leftover Lemon-Garlic Salmon and Asparagus	Ginger-Carrot Soup (page 156)	Milk-Boosting Granola (page 168) with reduced-fat milk
DAY 5	Leftover Creamiest Caramel Steel-Cut Oats	Leftover Ginger-Carrot Soup	Brisket with Prunes and Sweet Potatoes (page 164)	2 leftover Lactation Cookies, glass of reduced-fat milk or nondairy alternative
DAY 6	Quinoa Breakie Bowl (page 151)	Leftover Brisket with Prunes and Sweet Potatoes	Warming Sausage Soup (page 155)	Leftover Milk-Boosting Granola with reduced-fat milk
DAY 7	Avocado toast topped with 2 hard-boiled eggs and a sprinkle of red pepper flakes	Leftover Warming Sausage Soup with 1 apple	Winter Lentil Stew (page 158)	Chocolate almond butter with strawberries

Month 12 Sample Meal Plan

	BREAKFAST	LUNCH	DINNER	SNACK/ DESSERT
DAY 1	Chia-Berry Overnight Oats (page 149)	Roasted squash and root vegetable barley bowl with red cabbage and chopped dates	Ginger-Carrot Soup (page 156) with whole grain roll and green salad with vinegar and olive oil	Pineapple cubes with lime and mint and a handful of pistachios
DAY 2	Breakfast Sandwich (page 152) and ½ cup fresh berries	Leftover Ginger-Carrot Soup with whole grain roll	Scallop and Strawberry Salad (page 153)	2 Lactation Cookies (page 165) and a glass of reduced-fat milk
DAY 3	Leftover Chia-Berry Overnight Oats	Leftover Scallop and Strawberry Salad	Brisket with Prunes and Sweet Potato (page 164)	Nori sheets, avocado slices, and a sprinkle of sesame seeds
DAY 4	Quinoa Breakie Bowl (page 151)	Leftover Brisket with Prunes and Sweet Potato	Lemon-Garlic Salmon and Asparagus (page 163)	Air-popped popcorn sprinkled with nutritional yeast
DAY 5	Leftover Breakfast Sandwich with ½ cup fresh berries	Leftover Lemon-Garlic Salmon and Asparagus	Slow Cooker Chicken with Mango Salsa (page 162) with steamed veggies	Broiled Grapefruit with Frozen Yogurt and Crushed Brazil Nuts (page 166)
DAY 6	Pear, almond, and vanilla Greek yogurt parfait topped with Milk-Boosting Granola (page 168)	Wrap with leftover Slow Cooker Chicken with Mango Salsa and lettuce with 1 apple	Zucchini Noodles with Burst Cherry Tomatoes and Garlic (page 160)	Guacamole, salsa, and baked whole grain chips
DAY 7	Leftover Breakfast Sandwich with 1 cup chopped cantaloupe	Leftover Zucchini Noodles with Burst Cherry Tomatoes and Garlic	Bone Broth Ramen (page 159)	Leftover Broiled Grapefruit with Frozen Yogurt and Crushed Brazil Nuts

Chia-Berry Overnight Oats

VEGETARIAN

SERVES 4

PREP TIME: 2 minutes, plus 4 hours chill time

Chia seeds have a unique balance of insoluble and soluble fiber, so they are a magical addition to your diet for bowel health, helping with both loose and hard stools both before and after baby comes. Chia seeds are also a fantastic prebiotic, meaning their fiber feeds the good bacteria in your digestive tract.

1¼ cups full-fat coconut milk

1 cup rolled oats

½ cup blueberries

¼ cup plain whole-milk yogurt

2 tablespoons chia seeds

2 tablespoons almond butter

¼ teaspoon pure vanilla extract or vanilla bean powder

Dash cinnamon

1. In a medium bowl, combine the coconut milk, oats, blueberries, yogurt, chia seeds, almond butter, vanilla, and cinnamon. Stir well.

2. Divide the mixture into airtight containers and refrigerate for at least 4 hours or overnight.

Ingredient tip: If you are avoiding dairy, choose coconut yogurt. Or, omit the yogurt and add a ¼ cup more of coconut milk and ½ teaspoon of probiotic powder. For a warm breakfast, cook all the ingredients in a small pot over low heat until warm. For a grain-free option, omit the oats and double the chia seeds.

Per serving: Calories: 380; Total Fat: 26g; Saturated Fat: 16g; Cholesterol: 0mg; Sodium: 25mg; Carbohydrates: 28g; Fiber: 8g; Protein: 8g

Creamiest Caramel Steel-Cut Oats

DAIRY-FREE, VEGETARIAN

SERVES 4

PREP TIME: 5 minutes / **COOK TIME:** 40 minutes

Steel-cut oats are the least-processed form of oats you can buy at the grocery store, which means they have the most fiber. Oats contain a carbohydrate called beta-glucan that prevents abrupt increases in blood sugar levels after you eat it. Including full-fat coconut milk will also help keep your blood sugar stable, which is another way this easy breakfast supports you in these first postpartum months.

½ cup full-fat coconut milk

1½ cups water

¼ cup pure maple syrup

1 tablespoon coconut oil

1 teaspoon pure vanilla extract or vanilla bean powder

¼ teaspoon salt

1 cup steel-cut oats

1. In a medium pot, stir together the coconut milk and water over high heat and bring to a boil. Add the maple syrup, coconut oil, vanilla, and salt and stir well to combine.

2. Add the oats to the pot and stir well. Reduce the heat to low, cover, and cook for 35 minutes, stirring occasionally to ensure the bottom is not burning.

3. Spoon into bowls and serve hot.

Storage tip: Store leftovers in an airtight container in the refrigerator for up to 1 week or in the freezer for up to 6 months. To reheat, cook with a little extra water over low heat, stirring frequently, until hot.

Per serving: Calories: 330; Total Fat: 15g; Saturated Fat: 11g; Cholesterol: 0mg; Sodium: 135mg; Carbohydrates: 39g; Fiber: 5g; Protein: 6g

Quinoa Breakie Bowl

GLUTEN-FREE, NUT-FREE, VEGETARIAN

SERVES 2

PREP TIME: 5 minutes / **COOK TIME:** 10 minutes

This is a breakfast spin on a classic "fried" rice recipe, made with quinoa to lower the overall carbohydrate content. If you respond well to grains, feel free to make this with a whole grain like brown rice instead of quinoa. It's another great way to get some eggs in before noon, without them being the central focus. Although eggs are the prominent source of choline here, quinoa contains a little over 50mg per cooked cup as well.

1 tablespoon butter

½ yellow onion, chopped

2 garlic cloves, minced

¼ cup sweet corn

¼ cup peas

¼ cup shredded carrots

1 cup cooked quinoa

2 large eggs

¼ teaspoon salt

Freshly ground black pepper

1. In a medium pan, heat the butter over medium heat. Add the onion and garlic and cook for 5 minutes until softened.

2. Add the corn, peas, and carrot and continue to cook for 5 minutes, stirring occasionally.

3. Add the quinoa, breaking it up with a spoon as you stir. As it begins to soften, add the eggs and continue to stir until thoroughly cooked.

4. Season with the salt and pepper and serve immediately.

Ingredient tip: Day-old cooked quinoa has a better consistency for this dish than moist, freshly made quinoa. Saving quinoa from a previous dinner is the perfect way to have it on hand to stir up this breakfast dish in minutes.

Per serving: Calories: 337; Total Fat: 19g; Saturated Fat: 6g; Cholesterol: 179mg; Sodium: 318mg; Carbohydrates: 31g; Fiber: 5g; Protein: 12g

Breakfast Sandwiches

NUT-FREE, FREEZER-FRIENDLY

SERVES 6

PREP TIME: 5 minutes / **COOK TIME:** 25 minutes

Make these sandwiches before baby arrives or when you have a free moment for busy mornings. Not only will the egg give you protein to get your day started, but eggs also contain choline, which is essential for your baby's brain development. Serve with a side of fruit, such as berries that contain vitamin C, potassium, folate, and fiber.

Nonstick cooking spray

10 large eggs

1 cup whole milk

Pinch salt

6 whole grain English muffins

6 nitrite-free turkey sausage patties or bacon slices

6 slices cheese of choice

1. Preheat the oven to 375°F. Prepare three baking sheets with cooking spray.

2. In a large mixing bowl, beat together the eggs, milk, and salt. Once combined, pour this mixture gently into one of the baking sheets. Place in the oven and set a timer for 10 minutes.

3. Prep the English muffins by cutting them in half and placing them, cut-side up, on another baking sheet. Place the sausage patties onto the final baking sheet.

4. After 10 minutes has passed, add the sausage patties to the oven. Check on the eggs, which should still need another 10 to 15 minutes. Set another timer for 5 minutes.

5. After 5 minutes has passed, add the English muffins to the oven and allow everything to cook for 5 more minutes.

6. Remove all three baking sheets and prep a surface for assembly. Cut the egg mixture into six squares. Assemble the sandwiches by placing one half of the English muffin first, followed by the egg, a slice of cheese, a sausage patty, and the other half of the English muffin. Wrap in foil and place in freezer.

7. To reheat, remove the foil, wrap in damp paper towel, and microwave for 2 minutes on 50 percent power.

Per serving: Calories: 424; Total Fat: 22g; Saturated Fat: 8g; Cholesterol: 361mg; Sodium: 688mg; Carbohydrates: 30g; Fiber: 2g; Protein: 26g

Scallop and Strawberry Salad

GLUTEN-FREE

SERVES 4

PREP TIME: 5 minutes / **COOK TIME:** 6 minutes

The combination of the sweet strawberries and candied pecans with the citrus-flavored scallops makes for a refreshing taste in this salad. Although some seafoods contain high levels of mercury, scallops are not only safe to eat, but also recommended! Fresh straw- berries are also excellent both during and after pregnancy, thanks to their high vitamin C content.

4 cups spring lettuce mix

1 cup sliced strawberries

½ cucumber, sliced

¼ cup candied pecans

3 tablespoons balsamic
  vinaigrette, divided

¼ cup butter

2 garlic cloves, minced

8 sea scallops

Juice of ½ lemon

1. In a large bowl, toss the lettuce, strawberries, cucumber, pecans, and 2 tablespoons of vinaigrette and set aside.

2. In a large skillet, heat the butter and garlic over medium-high heat. Swirl the pan until the butter is melted and browned.

3. Add the scallops to the pan. Cook for the 3 minutes, then gently flip and cook for an additional 3 minutes before removing from the pan.

4. Split the salad into four portions, creating a bed for the scallops.

5. Squeeze the lemon over the cooked scallops and gently place 2 scallops on each salad. Top with the remaining tablespoon of vinaigrette and serve.

Cooking tip: When cooking the scallops, be sure to leave plenty of room around each one. This will create the optimal temperature for proper searing.

Per serving: Calories: 265; Total Fat: 20g; Saturated Fat: 8g; Cholesterol: 48mg; Sodium: 348mg; Carbohydrates: 11g; Fiber: 2g; Protein: 12g

Lemon, Arugula, and Quinoa Salad

GLUTEN-FREE, VEGETARIAN

SERVES 6

PREP TIME: 10 minutes / **COOK TIME:** 15 minutes

Pseudo-grains like quinoa, while still on the starchy side, are actually seeds, and they incorporate more protein and fiber into their structure than other true grains such as rice. This means there is a less negative effect on your blood sugar when you eat them. I also included peppery arugula in this recipe for two reasons. One, it's sturdy enough to hold together long enough to be eaten as a leftover. Two, it adds calcium, vitamin A, folate, magnesium, and choline.

1 cup quinoa, rinsed and drained

2 cups Slow Cooker Beef Bone Broth (page 87)

8 cups arugula

1 avocado, pitted, peeled, and chopped

1 cup cherry tomatoes, halved

½ cup slivered almonds

½ cup crumbled feta cheese

¼ cup extra-virgin olive oil

3 tablespoons fresh lemon juice

½ teaspoon garlic powder

½ teaspoon dried oregano

Sea salt

Freshly ground black pepper

1. In a medium pan over medium-high heat, combine the quinoa and broth. Bring to a boil, cover, reduce the heat to low, and simmer for 15 minutes, until the broth is absorbed.

2. In a large bowl, toss together the arugula, avocado, tomatoes, almonds, and feta.

3. In a small bowl, whisk together the olive oil, lemon juice, garlic powder, oregano, salt, and pepper. Pour into the bowl with the arugula and toss to combine.

4. When the quinoa is cool, fluff it with a fork and mix into the salad.

5. Serve immediately.

Cooking tip: Using bone broth to cook grains or make soup adds significantly more protein (around 9 grams per cup) than regular broth.

Per serving: Calories: 328; Total Fat: 22g; Saturated Fat: 4g; Cholesterol: 11mg; Sodium: 247mg; Carbohydrates: 26g; Fiber: 6g; Protein: 11g

Warming Sausage Soup

DAIRY-FREE, GLUTEN-FREE

SERVES 6

PREP TIME: 10 minutes / **COOK TIME:** 30 minutes

As the recipe name lets on, the spices and ingredients in this superfood soup are warming to your digestion and satisfying to your soul. Their fiery, thermogenic properties literally warm your insides and aid digestion. Softened vegetables go easy on your stomach while gentle, healthy fats and proteins from the coconut milk and bone broth nourish and soothe the gut lining. If using store-bought broth, be aware of the potentially higher sodium content and consider not adding any more salt.

2½ tablespoons coconut oil

2 carrots, chopped

2 celery stalks, chopped

1 medium yellow onion, chopped

½ teaspoon salt

2 tablespoons curry powder

½ teaspoon ground ginger

1 pound chicken sausage, sliced

1 sweet potato, peeled and chopped

1 (15-ounce) can diced tomatoes

3 cups Slow Cooker Beef Bone Broth (page 87)

1 (13.5-ounce) can full-fat coconut milk

1 cup chopped fresh kale

2 tablespoons fresh lime juice

1. In a large pot over medium-high heat, heat the coconut oil. Add the carrot, celery, onion, and salt and cook for 5 minutes, stirring occasionally, until softened. Add the curry powder and ginger and stir to incorporate.

2. Add the sausage and cook for 5 minutes, breaking it up with a spoon as it cooks.

3. Add the sweet potato and tomatoes with their juices and cook for another 5 minutes. Add the broth, coconut milk, and kale, bring the mixture to a simmer, and cook for 20 minutes.

4. Just before serving, stir in the lime juice. Spoon into bowls and serve.

Cooking tip: For a thicker soup, use an immersion blender to puree some of the soup until it reaches a creamier consistency.

Per serving: Calories: 400; Total Fat: 29g; Saturated Fat: 22g; Cholesterol: 23mg; Sodium: 600mg; Carbohydrates: 20g; Fiber: 5g; Protein: 18g

Ginger-Carrot Soup

DAIRY-FREE, GLUTEN-FREE

SERVES 6

PREP TIME: 10 minutes / **COOK TIME:** 20 minutes

Turmeric is a powerful uterotonic herb that reduces postpartum hemorrhage and ginger supports breast milk production. If using store-bought broth, be aware of the potentially higher sodium content and consider not adding any more salt.

1 tablespoon coconut oil

1 yellow onion, chopped

2 garlic cloves, minced

1 pound carrots, peeled and chopped

1½ tablespoons minced fresh ginger

½ teaspoon ground turmeric

4 cups Slow Cooker Beef Bone Broth (page 87) or store-bought

1 (13.5-ounce) can coconut milk

½ teaspoon salt

Freshly ground black pepper

1 tablespoon fresh lime juice

2 tablespoons sesame seeds

1. In a large soup pot, melt the coconut oil over medium heat. Add the onion and garlic and stir for 2 minutes.

2. Add the carrot, ginger, and turmeric and cook for about 5 minutes, until the carrots begin to soften.

3. Add the broth, coconut milk, salt, and pepper, stir once, and simmer for 15 minutes.

4. Take the pan off the heat and stir in the lime juice.

5. Transfer the soup to a blender in batches and blend until smooth.

6. Spoon into bowls, garnish with sesame seeds, and serve immediately.

Cooking tip: To make this soup vegetarian, swap out the bone broth for vegetable broth. When using a blender to puree the hot soup, blend in small batches and never fully close the lid. You can remove the plug in the blender lid and place a clean dish towel over the top to allow steam to escape without letting the soup splash out.

Per serving: Calories: 265; Total Fat: 21g; Saturated Fat: 17g; Cholesterol: 0mg; Sodium: 445mg; Carbohydrates: 17g; Fiber: 4g; Protein: 6g

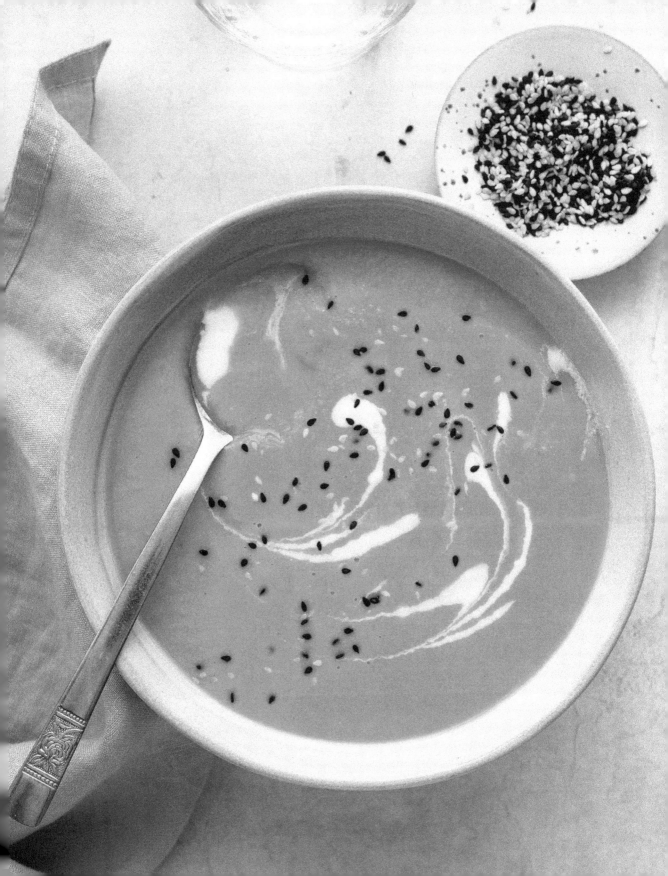

Winter Lentil Stew

GLUTEN-FREE, FREEZER-FRIENDLY

SERVES 6

PREP TIME: 10 minutes / **COOK TIME:** 30 minutes

Lentils are a fantastic and often untapped source of fiber and folate. I throw in a handful of finely chopped spinach to most of my soups and stews because it's an easy way to get a big hit of vitamin K, beta-carotene, folate, magnesium, and non-heme iron. For a vegetarian recipe, swap out the bone broth for vegetable broth.

2 tablespoons butter

1 sweet onion, chopped

5 carrots, peeled and chopped

3 celery stalks, minced

1½ teaspoons garlic powder

6 cups Slow Cooker Beef Bone Broth
  (page 87) or store-bought

2 pounds sweet potatoes, peeled
  and cubed

1 cup brown lentils

1 cup finely chopped fresh spinach

2 tablespoons Dijon mustard

2 tablespoons coconut aminos

1 teaspoon dried basil

½ teaspoon dried thyme

½ teaspoon salt

1. In a large pot, melt the butter over medium heat, then add the onion, carrot, celery, and garlic powder and stir to combine. Cook for 5 minutes until softened.

2. Add the broth, sweet potatoes, lentils, spinach, mustard, coconut aminos, basil, thyme, and salt and stir to combine. Adjust the heat to medium-high, cover and bring to a boil. Immediately reduce the heat to low and simmer for 25 minutes, until the lentils and sweet potatoes are tender.

3. Spoon into bowls and serve.

Cooking tip: If you'd like a thicker stew, use an immersion blender to blend small portions of the vegetables. Alternatively, mash some of the sweet potatoes with a fork.

Per serving: Calories: 401; Total Fat: 5g; Saturated Fat: 3g; Cholesterol: 10mg; Sodium: 503mg; Carbohydrates: 58g; Fiber: 10g; Protein: 31g

Bone Broth Ramen

DAIRY-FREE, NUT-FREE

SERVES 4

PREP TIME: 10 minutes / **COOK TIME:** 20 minutes

You no longer have to rely on restaurants for good ramen. This recipe is extremely easy, with the most difficult step being to find these ingredients in the specialty section of your grocery store. Bone broth is rich in important amino acids that can help support post-partum healing. Seaweed gives this soup a boost of iodine, a key nutrient during lactation. To top it all off, this hearty ramen is garnished with a hard-boiled egg for an extra source of protein and choline.

1 (8-ounce) package whole wheat soba noodles

4 cups pastured Slow Cooker Beef Bone Broth (page 87) or store-bought

1 cup sliced shiitake mushrooms

4 nori sheets, cut into strips

4 garlic cloves, minced

1 tablespoon minced fresh ginger

Salt

4 scallions, both white and green parts, chopped

4 hard-boiled eggs, peeled and halved

1. Bring a large pot of water to a boil and cook the soba noodles according to the package directions. Once cooked, drain, rinse, and set aside.

2. In a large pot, heat the bone broth over medium-high heat. Once boiling, reduce to a simmer and add the mushrooms, nori, garlic, and ginger. Cover and cook for 3 minutes.

3. Taste and add salt as needed. Once the seaweed is wilted, pour the broth into four bowls. Divide the noodles among the bowls and garnish each with scallions and an egg.

Substitution tip: To make this dish gluten-free, opt for buckwheat noodles. Add a variety of vegetables like carrots and bok choy for extra nutrients.

Per serving: Calories: 318; Total Fat: 6g; Saturated Fat: 2g; Cholesterol: 164mg; Sodium: 526mg; Carbohydrates: 49g; Fiber: 2g; Protein: 22g

Zucchini Noodles with Burst Cherry Tomatoes and Garlic

GLUTEN-FREE, NUT-FREE

SERVES 4

PREP TIME: 10 minutes / **COOK TIME:** 10 minutes

Zucchini noodles (aka zoodles) are a great alternative to pasta made from simple carbohydrates. If you don't own a spiralizer, use a vegetable peeler to create long ribbons. Chicken sausage is a lean protein choice that will fuel your body in this simple veggie-forward dish.

2 tablespoons ghee

1 cup cherry tomatoes, halved

2 garlic cloves, minced

2 pounds cooked chicken sausage, cut into coins

2 medium zucchini, spiralized

Sea salt

Freshly ground black pepper

1. In a skillet, melt the ghee over medium heat. Add the tomatoes and garlic and cook for 5 minutes, until the tomatoes have started to burst. Add the sausage and cook for another 2 minutes.

2. Add the zucchini noodles and cook for about 2 minutes, until just softened. Season with salt and pepper.

3. Serve immediately.

Ingredient tip: Zucchini noodles have a tendency to become soggy and fall apart if cooked for too long. Err on the side of undercooking your zoodles.

Per serving: Calories: 503; Total Fat: 25g; Saturated Fat: 9g; Cholesterol: 202mg; Sodium: 1,356mg; Carbohydrates: 24g; Fiber: 4g; Protein: 44g

Chicken Thigh Tzatziki Bowls

GLUTEN-FREE, NUT-FREE

SERVES 4

PREP TIME: 10 minutes, plus 10 minutes to 6 hours chill time / **COOK TIME:** 20 minutes

Traditional tzatziki sauce beautifully features probiotic-rich yogurt in a savory dish, which can be hard to find. Plain yogurt boasts vitamins A, B$_{12}$, and K$_2$, iodine, zinc, and calcium, not to mention high levels of protein and good fat. Before cooking the chicken, soak four bamboo skewers in water for at least 30 minutes (or overnight).

1 teaspoon extra-virgin olive oil

½ tablespoon red wine vinegar

½ teaspoon dried oregano

½ teaspoon salt

1 pound boneless chicken thighs, cut into 1-inch pieces

1 cup grated cucumber

½ cup plain Greek yogurt

1 teaspoon fresh lemon juice

½ teaspoon dried dill or 1 tablespoon minced fresh dill

¼ teaspoon garlic powder

2 cups cooked quinoa

1 cup cherry tomatoes, diced

1 cup pitted green olives

¼ cup sliced red onion

¼ cup crumbled feta cheese

1. In a large bowl, mix the olive oil, vinegar, oregano, and salt to make a marinade. Add the chicken and mix until entirely covered. Cover the bowl and refrigerate for at least 10 minutes or up to 6 hours.

2. Set a cast-iron skillet over medium-high heat. Thread the chicken onto four bamboo skewers. Discard the marinade. Cook the skewers in the skillet, turning occasionally, until cooked through, about 15 minutes.

3. In a small bowl, mix together the cucumber, yogurt, lemon juice, dill, and garlic powder.

4. Divide the quinoa, tomatoes, olives, and onion evenly among four bowls. Place a chicken skewer on top of each bowl, dollop with the tzatziki, and sprinkle with feta.

Cooking tip: To remove excess moisture from the shredded cucumber, press it between layers of paper towels before adding to the tzatziki.

Per serving: Calories: 517; Total Fat: 30g; Saturated Fat: 8g; Cholesterol: 160mg; Sodium: 1,490mg; Carbohydrates: 29g; Fiber: 4g; Protein: 30g

Slow Cooker Chicken with Mango Salsa

DAIRY-FREE, GLUTEN-FREE, NUT-FREE

SERVES 4

PREP TIME: 15 minutes / **COOK TIME:** 5 hours

The best thing about this recipe is how easy it is, thanks to your slow cooker. Combining chicken with vitamin C–rich foods like red bell pepper supports your body's healing. This recipe is also packed with fiber to keep constipation at bay.

2 ripe mangoes, peeled, cored, and chopped

1 small red onion, chopped

½ cup chopped fresh cilantro

½ cup brown sugar

1 jalapeño, seeded and finely chopped

Juice of 1 lime

4 boneless, skinless chicken breasts

1 red bell pepper, thinly sliced

1 tablespoon salt

1. In a large bowl, combine the mango, onion, cilantro, brown sugar, jalapeño, and lime juice.

2. Place the chicken breasts in the slow cooker and pour the mango mixture over the chicken. Add the bell pepper and the salt.

3. Cover and cook on high for 5 hours or until fully cooked.

4. Shred the chicken with a fork and serve over rice, as a taco filler, or however else you wish to enjoy.

Cooking tip: If you don't have a slow cooker, follow the same instructions using a Dutch oven. Preheat the oven to 400°F and cook the chicken dish for 30 minutes, or until chicken is fully cooked.

Per serving: Calories: 319; Total Fat: 4g; Saturated Fat: 1g; Cholesterol: 80mg; Sodium: 1,828mg; Carbohydrates: 48g; Fiber: 4g; Protein: 27g

DAIRY-FREE, GLUTEN-FREE, NUT-FREE

SERVES 4

PREP TIME: 10 minutes / **COOK TIME:** 20 minutes

Salmon is a low-mercury fish bursting with nutrients such as calcium, vitamin D, omega-3s, B$_{12}$*, vitamin A, and choline. Calcium is critical for breastfeeding, and salmon has just what you need!*

1½ pounds wild-caught salmon, cut into 4 pieces

2 pounds asparagus, trimmed

½ red onion, sliced

3 tablespoons extra-virgin olive oil

1½ tablespoons fresh lemon juice

4 garlic cloves, minced

1 teaspoon Dijon mustard

½ teaspoon salt

¼ teaspoon freshly ground black pepper

1. Preheat the oven to 400°F. Prepare a rimmed baking sheet and four (5-inch) squares of parchment paper.

2. Place a piece of salmon in the center of each of the pieces of parchment paper. Arrange some of the asparagus and onion around each fish.

3. In a small bowl, combine the olive oil, lemon juice, garlic, mustard, salt, and pepper. Divide equally among the salmon and vegetables. Close up the parchment paper and place on the baking sheet.

4. Bake for 10 minutes. Carefully open the parchment paper and toss the vegetables. Rewrap the parchment paper and return to the oven, checking every 5 minutes until the salmon is cooked and the vegetables reach your desired doneness.

Cooking tip: To create parchment packets, place the fish in the center of your parchment sheet. Add any other ingredients. Fold the parchment paper by bringing the two ends to the center and crimping to close the package. Then roll the two remaining sides toward the center and crimp to seal.

Per serving: Calories: 356; Total Fat: 17g; Saturated Fat: 3g; Cholesterol: 125mg; Sodium: 344mg; Carbohydrates: 12g; Fiber: 5g; Protein: 40g

Brisket with Prunes and Sweet Potatoes

DAIRY-FREE, GLUTEN-FREE, NUT-FREE, FREEZER-FRIENDLY

SERVES 6

PREP TIME: 30 minutes / **COOK TIME:** 5 hours 10 minutes

This brisket is loaded with iron and zinc, two nutrients that are essential during the post-partum period. If you are breastfeeding, the sweet potatoes in this dish will fuel your body with beta carotene, which will be converted to vitamin A in your body. Because vitamin A needs increase during lactation, this is a perfect dinner to help meet your quota. This dish is easily freezable and is a wonderful option to prepare before baby arrives.

3 tablespoons extra-virgin olive oil

4½ pounds beef brisket

3 large yellow onions, diced

5 garlic cloves, thinly sliced

Salt

2 cups beef broth

1 cup pitted prunes

2 sweet potatoes, peeled and diced

1. Preheat the oven to 300°F. Prepare a large roasting pan by heating the olive oil in over medium-high heat.

2. Place the brisket into the pan, fat-side down. Cook for about 10 minutes, turning once, until the fat renders. Once cooked, remove the brisket from the pan and set aside.

3. Place the onion and garlic in the hot pan and stir well. Add the brisket back to the pan, fat-side up, and season with salt. Cover and bake in the oven for 2 hours.

4. After 2 hours, add the beef broth and prunes, re-cover, and bake for another hour and a half.

5. Add the sweet potatoes to the pot, cover, and cook for another 30 minutes, or until the potatoes are tender.

6. Let stand for 30 minutes before removing the contents of the pot and basting the meat in the cooking liquid. Cut the meat against the grain and serve.

Cooking tip: You can prepare this dish in a slow cooker, too. Cook for at least 6 hours on low heat, or until cooked to your liking.

Per serving: Calories: 731; Total Fat: 32g; Saturated Fat: 10g; Cholesterol: 211mg; Sodium: 547mg; Carbohydrates: 35g; Fiber: 5g; Protein: 74g

Lactation Cookies

DAIRY-FREE, FREEZER-FRIENDLY, NUT-FREE, VEGETARIAN

MAKES 20 COOKIES

PREP TIME: 15 minutes / **COOK TIME:** 10 minutes

If you are breastfeeding, lactation cookies are a wonderful way to get galactagogues, or items that are thought to promote breast milk production, into your diet. These cookies are an easy snack to pop into your mouth on busy days when you need a boost.

½ cup water

¼ cup ground flaxseed

1 cup coconut sugar

⅓ cup melted coconut oil

¼ cup debittered brewer's yeast

1 teaspoon vanilla extract

½ teaspoon baking soda

¼ teaspoon salt

2 cups oat flour

¾ cup rolled oats

⅔ cup dairy-free dark chocolate chips

1. Preheat the oven to 350°F. Line a baking sheet with parchment paper.

2. In a large bowl, combine the water and flaxseed and set aside for 5 minutes to create a "flax egg."

3. After 5 minutes has passed, add the coconut sugar, coconut oil, brewer's yeast, vanilla, baking soda, and salt to the flax egg.

4. Once thoroughly combined, gradually add the rolled oats until a dough is formed. Fold in the oats and dark chocolate chips.

5. Drop the dough onto the parchment paper in spoonfuls, about 2 inches apart, and use a fork to flatten them.

6. Bake for 12 minutes, until lightly golden on top.

7. Let cool before eating. Store in an airtight container at room temperature for up to 1 week.

Prep tip: Before baby is born, premake the dough and freeze in individual portions. When you want a fresh cookie, defrost the desired quantity of dough and bake. If you are not avoiding dairy, feel free to use whichever chocolate chips you desire.

Per serving (1 cookie): Calories: 171; Total Fat: 7g; Saturated Fat: 4g; Cholesterol: 1mg; Sodium: 68mg; Carbohydrates: 25g; Fiber: 3g; Protein: 4g

Broiled Grapefruit with Frozen Yogurt and Crushed Brazil Nuts

GLUTEN-FREE, VEGETARIAN

SERVES 4

PREP TIME: 10 minutes / **COOK TIME:** 15 minutes

Grapefruit are loaded with breastmilk-boosting nutrients and are naturally refreshing, hydrating, and satisfying as you recover after baby is born. The addition of Brazil nuts gives this dish a protein boost along with a dose of selenium, a nutrient that is needed in sufficient amounts when breastfeeding.

2 large grapefruits, halved crosswise

1 cup crushed Brazil nuts

½ cup brown sugar

2 tablespoons unsalted butter, melted

1 teaspoon ground cinnamon

2 cups vanilla frozen yogurt

1. Preheat the broiler to 425°F.

2. In a baking dish, place the grapefruit halves, cut-side up, in the dish.

3. In a small bowl, combine the nuts, brown sugar, butter, and cinnamon. Sprinkle the mixture evenly over the flesh side of the grapefruit halves. Broil for 2 to 3 minutes, until the sugar is bubbly. Remove from the heat.

4. Top each piece with ½ cup of vanilla frozen yogurt.

Substitution tip: Swap crushed almonds for Brazil nuts if you prefer. To make this dish dairy-free, use melted coconut oil in place of the butter and choose a coconut-based topping in place of the yogurt. Feel free to use oranges if there is any drug-nutrient concern.

Per serving: Calories: 521; Total Fat: 31g; Saturated Fat: 11g; Cholesterol: 27mg; Sodium: 62mg; Carbohydrates: 59g; Fiber: 6g; Protein: 9g

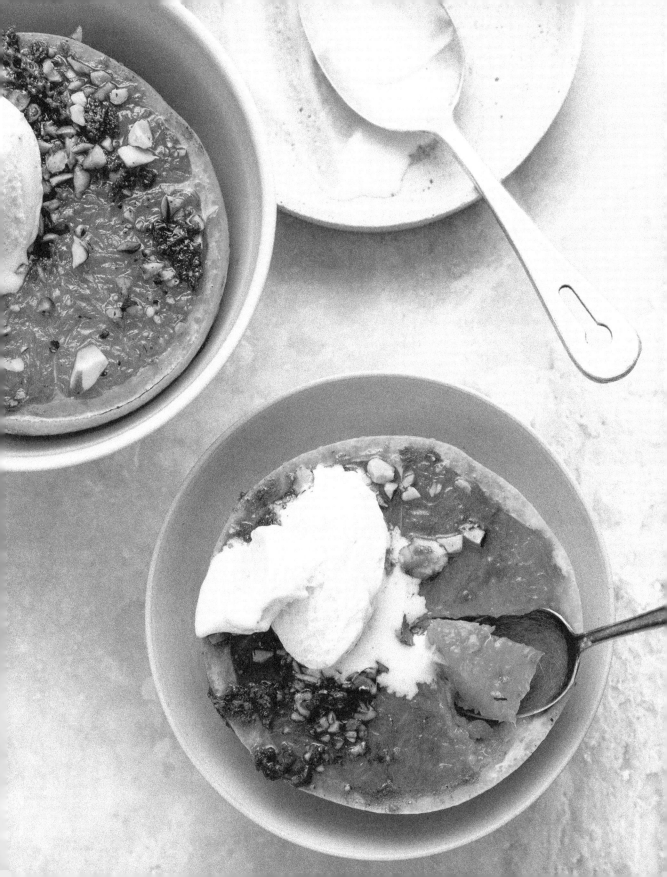

Milk-Boosting Granola

VEGETARIAN

SERVES 6

PREP TIME: 5 minutes / **COOK TIME:** 30 minutes

Granola is not only fun to make, but ridiculously easy, and this recipe is full of nutrients for you and baby. Oats can help prevent constipation because of their high fiber content. Although we need more data to say this definitively, many people lean on oats to help support a healthy milk supply. If you are not an oatmeal fan, granola is the next best thing to get this milk-boosting food into your diet.

2 cups rolled oats

½ cup chopped walnuts

½ cup slivered almonds

2 teaspoons ground cinnamon

½ teaspoon salt

¼ cup pure maple syrup

2 tablespoons melted coconut oil

2 tablespoons nut butter

½ cup chocolate chips

1. Preheat the oven to 300°F and line a large baking sheet with parchment paper.

2. In a large bowl, mix the oats, walnuts, almonds, cinnamon, and salt. Drizzle in the maple syrup and coconut oil. Add the nut butter and mix well.

3. Scoop the mixture onto the prepared baking sheet and form an oval shape. Press the mixture firmly down. Bake for 15 minutes.

4. Remove the baking sheet from the oven and rotate the pan. Break up the granola with a fork, but not so much that you disrupt any clumping.

5. Return the baking sheet to the oven and bake for another 15 minutes or until golden brown.

6. Let the granola cool for at least 20 minutes. Once it is fully cooled, break it up into pieces and add the chocolate chips. Enjoy!

Substitution tip: This recipe is fully customizable. Add your favorite nuts, nut butter, seeds, dried fruit, you name it! Store the granola in an airtight container for up to 1 month.

Per serving: Calories: 416; Total Fat: 25g; Saturated Fat: 8g; Cholesterol: 4mg; Sodium: 213mg; Carbohydrates: 41g; Fiber: 6g; Protein: 10g

MEASUREMENT CONVERSIONS

VOLUME EQUIVALENTS	US STANDARD	US STANDARD (OUNCES)	METRIC (APPROXIMATE)
LIQUID	2 tablespoons	1 fl. oz.	30 mL
	¼ cup	2 fl. oz.	60 mL
	½ cup	4 fl. oz.	120 mL
	1 cup	8 fl. oz.	240 mL
	1½ cups	12 fl. oz.	355 mL
	2 cups or 1 pint	16 fl. oz.	475 mL
	4 cups or 1 quart	32 fl. oz.	1 L
	1 gallon	128 fl. oz.	4 L
DRY	⅛ teaspoon	–	0.5 mL
	¼ teaspoon	–	1 mL
	½ teaspoon	–	2 mL
	¾ teaspoon	–	4 mL
	1 teaspoon	–	5 mL
	1 tablespoon	–	15 mL
	¼ cup	–	59 mL
	⅓ cup	–	79 mL
	½ cup	–	118 mL
	⅔ cup	–	156 mL
	¾ cup	–	177 mL
	1 cup	–	235 mL
	2 cups or 1 pint	–	475 mL
	3 cups	–	700 mL
	4 cups or 1 quart	–	1 L
	½ gallon	–	2 L
	1 gallon	–	4 L

OVEN TEMPERATURES

FAHRENHEIT	CELSIUS (APPROXIMATE)
250°F	120°C
300°F	150°C
325°F	165°C
350°F	180°C
375°F	190°C
400°F	200°C
425°F	220°C
450°F	230°C

WEIGHT EQUIVALENTS

US STANDARD	METRIC (APPROXIMATE)
½ ounce	15 g
1 ounce	30 g
2 ounces	60 g
4 ounces	115 g
8 ounces	225 g
12 ounces	340 g
16 ounces or 1 pound	455 g

RESOURCES

Academy of Nutrition and Dietetics. "Eating Right During Pregnancy." EatRight.org/health/pregnancy/what-to-eat-when-expecting /eating-right-during-pregnancy.

The American College of Gynecology. "Morning Sickness." ACOG.org /patient-resources/faqs/pregnancy/morning-sickness-nausea-and-vomiting -of-pregnancy.

American Diabetes Association. "Gestational Diabetes and a Healthy Baby?" Diabetes.org/diabetes/gestational-diabetes.

Clark, Stephanie and Willow Jarosh. *Healthy, Happy Pregnancy Cookbook.* Atria Books, 2016.

Houston, Traci. *The Gestational Diabetes Cookbook & Meal Plan.* Rockbridge Press, 2019.

Licalzi, Diana and Kerry Benson. *Drinking for Two.* Blue Star Press, 2019.

March of Dimes. "Nutrition, Weight & Fitness." MarchOfDimes.org /pregnancy/nutrition-weight-and-fitness.aspx.

Nichols, Lily. *Real Food for Pregnancy.* Self-published, 2018.

US Food and Drug Administration. "Advice about Eating Fish for Women Who Are or Might Become Pregnant, Breastfeeding Mothers, and Young Children." FDA.gov/food/consumers/advice-about-eating-fish.

Wick, Myra. *Mayo Clinic Guide to a Healthy Pregnancy.* 2nd ed. Mayo Clinic Press, 2018.

REFERENCES

Abu-Ouf, Noran M, and Mohammed M. Jan. "The Impact of Maternal Iron Deficiency and Iron Deficiency Anemia on Child's Health." *Saudi Medical Journal* 36, no. 2 (2015): 146–149. doi: 10.15537/smj.2015.2.10289.

Braarud, Hanne Cecilie, Maria Wik Markhaus, Siv Skotheim, Kjell Morten Stormark, Livar Frøyland, Ingvild Eide Graff, and Marian Kjellevold. "Maternal DHA Status during Pregnancy Has a Positive Impact on Infant Problem Solving: A Norwegian Prospective Observation Study." *Nutrients* 10, no. 5 (April 24, 2018): 529. doi: 10.3390/nu10050529.

Carlson Susan E., John Colombo, Byron J. Gajewski, Kathleen M. Gustafson, David Mundy, John Yeast, Michael K. Georgieff, Lisa A. Markley, Elizabeth H. Kerling, and Jill Shaddy. "DHA Supplementation and Pregnancy Outcomes. *American Journal of Clinical Nutrition* 97, no. 4 (April 2013): 808–15. doi: 10.3945/ajcn.112.050021.

Chiefari, E., B. Arcidiacono, D. Foti, and A. Brunetti. "Gestational Diabetes Mellitus: An Updated Overview." *Journal of Endocrinological Investigation* 40, no. 9 (September 2017): 899–909. doi: 10.1007/s40618-016-0607-5.

Hoge, Axelle, Valentine Tabar, Anne-Françoise Donneau, Nadia Dardenne, Sylvie Degee, Marie Timmermans, Michelle Nisolle, Michèle Guillaume, and Vincenzo Castronovo. "Imbalance between Omega-6 and Omega-3 Polyunsaturated Fatty Acids in Early Pregnancy Is Predictive of Postpartum Depression in a Belgian Cohort." *Nutrients* 11, no. 4 (April 18, 2019): 876. doi: 10.3390/nu11040876.

Institute of Medicine (US) Standing Committee on the Scientific Evaluation of Dietary Reference Intakes and its Panel on Folate, Other B Vitamins, and Choline. *Dietary Reference Intakes for Thiamin, Riboflavin, Niacin, Vitamin B_6, Folate, Vitamin B_{12}, Pantothenic Acid, Biotin, and Choline.* Washington (DC): National Academies Press (US); 1998.

Korsmo, Hunter W., Zinyin Jiang, and Marie A. Caudill. "Choline: Exploring the Growing Science on Its Benefits for Moms and Babies." *Nutrients* 11, no. 8 (August 7, 2019): 1823. doi: 10.3390/nu11081823.

Al-Kuran, O., L Al-Mehaisen, H. Bawadi, S. Beitawi, and Z. Amarin. "The Effect of Late Pregnancy Consumption of Date Fruit on Labour and Delivery." *Journal of Obstetrics and Gynaecology* 31, no. 1 (2011): 29–31. doi: 10.3109/01443615.2010.522267.

Miller, James L., and Caroline Signore. "Neural Tube Defect Rates Before and After Food Fortification with Folic Acid." *Birth Defects Research Part A: Clinical and Molecular Teratology* 70, no. 11 (November 2004): 844–5. doi: 10.1002/bdra.20075.

Prentice, A. "Maternal Calcium Requirements during Pregnancy and Lactation." *American Journal of Clinical Nutrition* 59, suppl. 2 (February 1994): 477S-482S; discussion 482S-483S. doi: 10.1093/ajcn/59.2.477S.

Shah Prakesh S., and Arne Ohlsson. "Effects of Prenatal Multimicronutrient Supplementation on Pregnancy Outcomes: A Meta-analysis." *CMAJ* 180, no. 12 (June 9, 2009): E99–E108. doi: 10.1503/cmaj.081777.

Teucher, Birgit, Manuel Olivares, and Héctor Cori. "Enhancers of Iron Absorption: Ascorbic Acid and Other Organic Acids. *International Journal for Vitamin and Nutrition Research* 74, no. 6 (November 2004): 403–19. doi: 10.1024/0300-9831.74.6.403.

Zhao, Wei, Xinyu Li, Zinghai Xia, Zhengnan Gao, and Cheng Han. "Iodine Nutrition during Pregnancy: Past, Present, and Future." *Biological Trace Element Research* 188, no. 1 (March 2019): 196–207. doi: 10.1007/s12011-018-1502-z.

Zimmerman, Michael B., and Richard F. Hurrell. "Nutritional Iron Deficiency." *Lancet* 370, no. 9586 (August 11, 2007): 511–20. doi: 10.1016/S0140-6736(07)61235-5.

INDEX

ACKNOWLEDGMENTS

I would like to thank my mother for her support during the book writing process. This book would have never been completed without you. I also want to thank my editor, Myryah Irby, who helped guide me during the writing process. This resource will help so many people who are *eating for two*. I also want to thank Callisto for giving me this amazing opportunity to contribute to the resources available for the pregnant population. Thank you for believing in me.

I also have to thank my friend Courtney who acted as a sounding board throughout this process, my husband who was my "expert" taste-tester, and my Papa who has forever been my guiding light throughout my career.

ABOUT THE AUTHOR

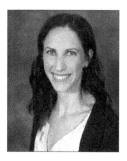

Lauren Manaker , MS, RDN, LDN, CLEC, CPT is an award-winning registered dietitian and certified lactation counselor-educator. After earning her bachelor of science degree from the University of Florida and her master of science degree from Rush University in Chicago, she has worked in the field of nutrition in hospital, office, and industry settings. Most recently, she works as a freelance writer and has been featured in outlets like CNN, *U.S. News & World Report*, and *EatingWell*. Lauren is an executive committee member of the Women's Health Dietetic Practice Group of the Academy of Nutrition and Dietetics. She has also authored fertility-related books and e-books and acts as an internship preceptor at the Medical University of South Carolina.

She also manages an Instagram account @fertility_prenatal_dietitian where she offers evidence-based tips for people who are trying to conceive or are currently pregnant. She resides in Charleston, South Carolina, with her daughter, husband, and rottweiler-chow mix.

ABOUT THE RECIPE DEVELOPER

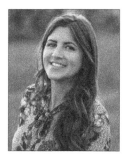

Madeline Given is a certified holistic nutritionist and mother, born and raised in Southern California. She's passionate about working alongside women, helping them find the freedom of health in their ever-changing bodies, from preconception through postpartum. She shares real food ideas for the whole family, with plenty of weaning and toddler ideas mixed in, on her Instagram (@madelinenutrition) and blog (MadelineNutrition.com).

CPSIA information can be obtained
at www.ICGtesting.com
Printed in the USA
JSHW031925310821
18232JS00001B/1